THE
HIDDEN
PLAGUE

A field guide for surviving & overcoming
hidradenitis suppurativa

TARA GRANT

THE HIDDEN PLAGUE

© 2013, Tara Grant

Library of Congress Control Number: 2013933723
Library of Congress Cataloging-in-Publication Data is on file with the publisher
Grant, Tara, 1974 –
The Hidden Plague / Tara Grant
ISBN: 978-1-939563-01-9
1. Health 2. Diet 3. Alternative therapies 4. Dermatology
Editor: Jessica Taylor Tudzin
Proofreader: Marion Warren
Indexer: Jeff Corral
Design and Layout: Caroline De Vita
Cover Design: Janée Meadows
Illustrations by Caroline De Vita, Virinaflora/Shutterstock.com, Ohmega1982/Shutterstock.com, and Potapov Alexander/Shutterstock.com

Publisher: Primal Blueprint Publishing.
23805 Stuart Ranch Rd. Suite 145 Malibu, CA 90265
For information on quantity discounts, please call 888-774-6259, email: info@primalblueprint.com, or visit PrimalBlueprintPublishing.com.

DISCLAIMER

I'm not a doctor. I don't have a degree in nutrition and I'm not a medically trained professional of any kind. I do, however, have some really cool traits: the ability to connect seemingly unrelated things and a basic understanding of some stuff in medical and nutrition journals. I visit doctors, read scientific studies, experiment on myself and then translate medical jargon into real words that are way more interesting to read than journals containing gobbledygook like "pro-inflammatory cytokines."

I have a degree in journalism from Carleton University in Canada—the top journalism school in the country. I am trained to report facts with an unbiased view. Any statistical data and specific scientific information I've included has been carefully researched, referenced, and checked for errors. I only use the work of research studies, books, and websites that have a reputation for accuracy and innovation. The people behind these sources are rock stars.

The advice in this book is not intended to diagnose or cure any disease. I provide details regarding my success at putting my own hidradenitis suppurativa into complete remission. It is up to you whether or not to implement these practices into your own self-treatment of the condition. These practices should not supersede nor conflict with instructions from your doctor. I cannot be held liable if you deviate from your doctor's counsel, advice, or prescription.

Current Western medical practice does not have a standard, effective treatment or cure for hidradenitis suppurativa or other autoimmune diseases and often suggests surgery or pharmaceutical intervention. Many medical professionals are also unaware of the existence and cause of HS. You should be aware of this.

I am required by law to inform you that you should always consult your doctor before starting anything new, whether it is a new diet or exercise regimen. I strongly advise that you visit a doctor before starting self-treatment to have tests done to rule out serious infections, including staph and MRSA. You also need to check with your doctor to see if a Primal or Paleolithic-style diet is right for you.

CONTENTS

FOREWORD

Howdy! My name is Robb Wolf. I'm a former research biochemist specializing in autoimmunity and cancer research. I also run a gym in Chico, California called NorCal Strength & Conditioning (One of *Mens Health*'s "Top 30 Gyms in America"). I've had the good fortune of pursuing a line of work that I not only love, but has helped millions of people. One of the people that I've been able to help is in fact the gorgeous author of the book you are now holding in your hands. Tara Grant has a fascinating story that is equal parts detective novel and self-transformation. She once suffered from myriad maladies, leaving her tired, lethargic, and, at certain points, hopeless. As is common for many people with non-typical health issues, Tara spent years just getting a solid diagnosis of what her condition was, which in this case was the autoimmune condition known as hidradenitis suppurativa (HS).

Autoimmunity is a process in which our body's own immune system attacks us. Normally the immune system protects us. It identifies a foreign invader (bacteria or virus), attacks it, and ideally clears the infection. All of us have molecules in our tissues that our immune system uses to recognize self from non-self, and this is where things can go haywire. For example, if a donated organ is not close enough to the recipient in tissue type, the immune system will attack and destroy the organ. In autoimmunity, a similar process occurs in that an individual's own tissue is confused as something foreign and the immune system attacks this "mislabeled" tissue.

Common forms of autoimmunity include multiple sclerosis, rheumatoid arthritis, lupus, and vitiligo, to name only a tiny fraction of autoimmune diseases. Elements of autoimmunity are likely at play in conditions as seemingly unrelated as schizophrenia, infertility, various forms of cancer, and hidradenitis suppurativa. Interestingly, all of these seemingly unrelated diseases share a common cause: damage to the intestinal lining which allows large, undigested food particles to make their way into the body. This is called *leaky gut and the autoimmune response.*

This may sound both scary and possibly familiar to you if you suffer from any type of autoimmune or systemic inflammatory condition. Lucky for you, however, because you have what may be the solution to a whole new way of life in your hands.

I've had many folks write to me about hidradenitis suppurativa, but Tara was the first to show that you can absolutely beat this thing with diet. She has pored through medical studies, found evidence linking HS to auto-immunity, and has managed to explain all the science mumbo-jumbo in a way that's easy to understand. For the first time, someone with this hor-rible condition has come forward and has not only exposed the suffering these people are going through, but has also given them concrete steps toward healing.

Something that is important to note up front: all autoimmune diseases, and a host of systemic inflammatory conditions (such as chronic fatigue), have what doctors call "common etiology" or "similar cause." Although this information is not widely known in mainstream medicine (yet) there are more and more doctors who are recommending what is called an *autoimmune paleo diet* to their patients suffering from these potentially life threatening conditions, and with remarkable success.

The paleo diet is the healthiest way you can eat because it is the only nutri-tional approach that works with your genetics to help you stay lean, strong, and energetic. Research indicates that our modern diet, full of refined foods, trans fats, and sugar, is at the root of degenerative diseases such as obesi-ty, cancer, diabetes, heart disease, Parkinson's, Alzheimer's, depression, and infertility, not to mention a host of other autoimmune conditions.

For most people, the fact the paleo diet delivers improved blood lipids, weight loss, and reduced pain from autoimmunity is proof enough. Many people, however, are not satisfied with blindly following any recommen-dations, be they nutrition or exercise related. Some folks need to know why they are doing something. Tara is one of these people. She has taken apart my autoimmune protocol step-by-step, added some other pertinent stuff with regards to HS, and put it all back together so that you can rid yourself of this disease for good. Oh, and I know most people are not swayed by silly sayings like "life saving" or "reversing disease"; we need something a bit more motivational like fitting into our skinny jeans. Not only will a paleo diet help you look great and feel fantastic, you will better your odds of living a long, long time to enjoy your newfound health.

If you're one of the millions of people affected by HS (or a host of other autoimmune problems), today is your lucky day.

Robb Wolf
Reno, Nevada
August 2013

The Lord will
strike you with
the same boils that
plagued the Egyptians.
He will strike you
with hemorrhoids,
sores, and itching that
won't go away.

—*Deuteronomy 28:27*

I didn't know the name of it

I have found a name for what I have been suffering

I feared I might be a msra carrier

I'm so embarrassed

I don't want anyone to find out

I'M ALWAYS IN PAIN

I'll do anything, ANYTHING

It is breaking my heart

I HAVEN'T TOLD ANYONE ELSE

I feel like I've tried everything

OMG! I'm in tears just knowing that someone is actually going to tell me
SOMETHING that might help

Reading this was like reading my life story

I am just miserable and self-conscious

I PRAY THIS WORKS. IT COULD BE LIFE-CHANGING

I believe that diet has helped me tremendously

I can get this under control   **YOU HAVE GIVEN ME HOPE**

Thank you... there will never be enough words

Thank you so much for giving us a voice

I know it can get better

THANK YOU. THANK YOU. THANK YOU. THANK YOU.

WELCOME

No doubt everything you've ever read on hidradenitis suppurativa (HS) has been depressing. Why? Because until now there have been few answers and little, if any, help. Many readers of PrimalGirl.com have said that my blog posts on this issue were the first real and helpful information they've received about their HS, probably because it comes from someone who understands the agony and embarrassment, the drive to end this scourge once and for all.

The comments on the opposite page are from readers just like you. Perhaps you have said many of these things yourself in your quest to find help. I know how desperate you are. I get you, more than people who don't have hidradenitis suppurativa ever will. I have survived this and you can too.

You may have hardened yourself to the possibility that this will never go away, that you will always live in pain and agony. To overcome HS, you need to become an advocate of your own health. You need to care. You need to take back your power. You need to want a better life. If you are willing to take ownership and make changes, and you are not willing to lie down and take it anymore, this book is for you. If, however, you have a victim mentality, be forewarned: I'm not willing to live like a victim and I don't write for them either.

You may find a few curse words thrown in now and then in the pages of this book. I've been accused of having a potty mouth, and I tend to curse like a sailor in my personal life. But make no mistake: when I curse in my writing, I *mean* it. Sometimes, simply no other word will do.

Speaking of curse words, within the pages of this book, you are going to find a detailed field guide for navigating the shitty, shitty hand you've been dealt. Since I'm not a doctor, I can't legally give you medical advice, so instead I will ...

- cite tons of references
- tell you everything I've learned
- tell you of my experiments and reactions
- tell you how I took care of my wounds
- tell you exactly what experts in the paleo community believe causes HS
- tell you what I did to slam my HS into complete remission

What you do with this information is up to you. But I can tell you this: you sure will feel empowered when you find out that YOU hold the key to stopping the pain. There is no medication or surgery of any kind on this journey. No one to pay, nothing to buy, no side effects, or recovery from expensive, painful procedures. In fact, this book may be the very last thing you ever buy to treat your HS.

I found the best way to put HS into remission is to kick it old school—take it back to the last time human beings experienced an evolutionary change—and bypass all the modern misinformation about nutrition and disease.

The ancestral or Primal/paleo lifestyle mentioned in this book couldn't be simpler. It works because it is based on the foods that our bodies evolved on. Primal and paleo diets, also known as ancestral diets, consist of the foods that our Paleolithic ancestors ate: meat, fish, fowl, eggs, vegetables, nuts, and seeds. Modern and prepared foods are off the table.

Our ancestors led relatively disease-free lives, without any of the modern problems that plague us today. Heart disease, obesity, and diabetes were virtually unheard of. Even dental cavities were extremely rare. Prehistoric human beings were fit, lean, and healthy—all without lowfat diet foods, corporate gyms, and hand sanitizer. These people didn't just exist; they *thrived*.

For better or for worse, we are genetically identical to human beings who existed tens of thousands of years ago. Although technology and modern conveniences have changed our lives, our genes still expect certain inputs in order to function optimally. When we don't fulfill those inputs, we put ourselves at risk for modern diseases such as autoimmunity.

The *autoimmune paleo protocol* outlined in this book takes the concept of an ancestral diet one step further by removing not only the Neolithic foods that can disrupt your digestion, but also some Paleolithic foods, such as eggs. For some people, especially those with weak immunity, these foods can cause gut permeability and trigger HS. By carefully following this stricter form of Primal/paleo eating and testing for reactions to foods, you may see not only a complete remission of your HS, but other seemingly unrelated problems like dandruff or intestinal bowel syndrome.

KATELYNN'S STORY

I am fourteen years old. I have been suffering from HS since I was ten. I wasn't diagnosed until this past March because I've been too embarrassed to talk to my parents or doctor about this. I don't know if this is the right place to be contacting you about it, but I am struggling terribly with my HS.

Antibiotics are no longer working to control my condition, and I am desperate for any kind of relief. Talking to my parents doesn't do much. You can't discuss this kind of matter with someone who doesn't understand what it is like to feel the pain and embarrassment, when they don't understand what it is like to isolate yourself from the world because you are scared to let anyone see what's really wrong with you. I've had girls in my gym class bully me about it in the locker room, and friends that turned out not to be friends, tell people how disgusting I am, and how I have STD's. It's ruining my life. I need something, and I mean anything, to help me.

Katelynn, 14
Pennsylvania, USA

When I "went Primal" in 2009, I immediately saw a reduction in my HS flare-ups. I experienced some other radical changes too: I lost 100 pounds, my polycystic ovary syndrome (PCOS) went away, my hair grew back, and my joint pain and endometriosis were gone. I was no longer depressed all the time, and I didn't get itchy anymore. It was clear to me that my genes liked what I was doing.

When I moved toward an autoimmune diet, the rest of my problems resolved, including the HS. I can happily say that I don't have a single thing wrong with me at the moment. I don't have a complaint in the world. But it wasn't always this way.

I've had HS since puberty. I started getting little pimples and bumps on my bum. I thought it was a normal part of growing up, just "teenage acne." I didn't tell anyone about it, except for my best friend at the time. She admitted that she got pimples on her bum too, which at the time served as further confirmation that this was all fairly normal.[1]

A couple years later I started getting the pimples in my groin area, except that they resembled boils more than pimples. The ones on my bum changed too. They were bigger and much more painful. When they erupted, out came pus, just like a pimple—only blood came out too. The boils took weeks to come to a head and months to heal. It was fairly common for another boil to pop up in the same place before the previous one had fully healed.

Of course, the boils left scars. Bad ones. If a boil didn't erupt, it would linger for months, leaving behind a dark spot when it finally did vanish. Other boils left pockmarks. They turned white after the angry purple scars faded away. And speaking of scars, they were every bit as emotional as they were physical.

For years, I didn't know anyone else who had this disease and I was too embarrassed to "come out." I felt alone and isolated. If I suspected that someone else might have it (there are telltale signs), I had to be the first to admit that I had it too. The disease damaged my self-esteem while I was growing up and limited the activities I was able to do.

Imagine a kid going through puberty, with all the stress and problems that puberty normally entails, and then add a frightening skin condition. Imagine going to a doctor and being told that it's caused by bacteria and the ensuing shame that comes from being told, "You aren't doing a good enough job of cleaning yourself. Down *there*." Imagine being told by countless doctors that they don't know what is wrong with you and that they don't have any solutions or treatments. All you know is that you're always ashamed and in pain.

Now imagine that *you* are that kid. Your friends are having a pool party. You really want to go but you are afraid that your bathing suit might ride up in the back and someone might see.

You don't go to that party, do you? You don't change in the locker room either. You don't go to sleepovers. You are afraid of being intimate. You think that people will think you are diseased, infected, contagious, damaged. Imagine the fragile self-esteem of a teenager who is afraid to reach out for help and who feels isolated and alone. It's hard having a secret.

I was that kid. Maybe you were too. I'm lucky that I had parents who constantly built me up, or God only knows how I may have turned out. Had I been raised in a strict religious family, I may have thought God had inflicted this disease upon me. After all, doesn't He punish people with boils from time to time, for some sin or another?

I'm lucky I didn't become obsessive-compulsive about keeping myself clean. Thinking that frequent scrubbing and cleansing would make the HS go away could have easily led to a disorder of some kind. Turns out, that kind of hygiene actually makes things worse, so I never really went too crazy in that direction.

The disease progressed slowly during my teens and early twenties. It was such a part of my life at that point that I figured I had to live with it. It was my cross to bear. I had a girlfriend in college who complained about a boil in her groin, so even then, I *still* thought all of this was fairly normal. My friend went to her doctor, was given antibiotics, and the boil cleared up. It's been years and I haven't checked in with this friend to see if the problem came back. I bet it did.

Over the years, my weight increased, as did my depression. Other symptoms—including irregular periods, cystic acne, allergies, hair loss, and recurrent infections—became a normal part of my life. The HS (or the "adult acne" as I thought of it then) got worse. I usually had about three boils at any given time. Convinced it was a form of acne, I started doing research and found a theory that tied acne to excessive sweating and bacteria. I also thought it might have something to do with ingrown hairs. Often, there was a hair trapped within the boil.

I was overweight, I did sweat more than the average person. I decided to shave off my pubic hair (against all the popular advice) to see if that would help and it actually did—I stopped getting flare-ups in my groin, but then got them worse on my behind. The problem simply migrated to a new area. Then I started getting horrible ingrown hairs—something I had never experienced before. I tried every remedy and cream on the market and nothing helped. I stopped shaving and the boils didn't come back to that area for about a year.

Some of my symptoms also cleared up when I went on birth control pills. But as HS is wont to do, it came back and continued unabated. Having a skin condition that looks like an STD on crack in your private areas—your groin, pubic area, buttocks, under your arms or breasts or anywhere you have hair follicles—will definitely affect how you interact with other people. HS trumped every other problem in my life.

When I went to my doctor, she told me I suffered from adult acne. Ha! She obviously didn't have a clue. I mentioned it a couple other times over the years to different doctors, but none of them could give me a name for the condition. They did reassure me they had seen it before and that I wasn't contagious.

None of the doctors I saw over the years understood autoimmunity and it's connection to the problem. No one ever gave me any sign of hope that this could get better. No one ever suggested perhaps it was something I was eating that was causing the outbreaks. I couldn't even find a doctor who knew the name of the disease! I struggled through my years with HS without the Internet, without support, without community.

Eventually, I started doing considerable research, found that my condition actually had a name, and started telling doctors what I had. I was immediately referred to a dermatologist.

After months of waiting to get an appointment, I walked out of the dermatologist's office after ten minutes with a firm diagnosis and the news that my only treatment option was a daily course of antibiotics. (I'll explain in later chapters why this treatment is more damaging than helpful.) I knew the dermatologist was wrong, and I knew that I actually knew more about HS than she did. I didn't take the pills; I was determined to find a natural cure.

It wasn't until I was in my mid-thirties and was already living a Primal lifestyle that I told my family about my HS. Growing up, I instinctively knew that if the doctors couldn't help, my parents—as loving and supportive as they were—wouldn't be able to either. Besides, my mom would have been beside herself with worry all those years. I just couldn't do that to her. I waited until I was able to put both a name and a treatment plan to the condition before opening up.

I have seen more than forty doctors from four different countries in my lifetime, and have gleaned three key concepts from them.

1. *Time.* Doctors don't have the time or the inclination to delve into a case like a detective. Real life is not like an episode of *House MD*.

2. *Blood Tests.* If the initial blood tests don't show anything, doctors are unlikely to look into the matter further.

3. ***Drugs.*** Doctors are more likely to recommend drugs than a change in diet.

This has been my experience, and from what I have heard from many of my readers, I'm not alone. I have learned that I have to be my own advocate when it comes to my health. No one else is going to do it for me. For twenty-five years, I have had to experiment on myself to treat my ailments. I've tried different pharmaceutical drugs, different diets, different exercise regimens, and followed the advice of various "experts."

For those of you who have seen doctors about this, I'm sorry. I'm betting about 90 percent of you have had a terrible experience. Only about 10 percent of the doctors I've seen in the last two decades seemed to have any interest in being kind and compassionate about what I was going through. (The doctors I saw specifically for HS are *not* included in this 10 percent.) Here are the things I was told over the years. I assume you have been given some similar advice:

1. You're not keeping yourself clean enough. Try using antibacterial soap, topical medications and wearing cotton underwear.

2. It's adult acne. We all get zits from time to time.

3. Don't shave. Keep your clothing loose. Don't wear a bra or anything that chafes against the area. Don't wear manmade materials.

4. Try not to sweat. It's your sweat glands doing this. Shower often to wash the bacteria off if you do sweat. Oh, and don't use deodorant.

5. We can incise the area, if you want, and drain it. That's your only option at this point.

6. Haven't you been taking the antibiotics I gave you? You know you need to take those every day for the rest of your life if you want to see improvement.

7. Try losing some weight. Oh, you have PCOS and one of the

symptoms is weight gain? Well, some of my patients have success with this if they lose weight. Just try to lose some. No, I don't know how.

"This is a life-long condition that you will have to live with," my dermatologist said. "There is no cure. The only treatment that has been shown to be effective in any way is a daily course of antibiotics. You will, of course, have to take them every day for the rest of your life. Until menopause, anyway. The disease usually 'burns itself out' at menopause."

I haven't seen or heard anything about HS "burning itself out" later in life in anything I've read, not even on the forums—just the occasional post-menopausal woman who seems to have the situation "under control," but still flares up occasionally. Perhaps she has it "under control" because she's been dealing with it for fifty years and has developed coping mechanisms. That doesn't sound like control to me—it sounds like denial.

Not one doctor asked me if this was interfering with my personal relationships, if it was screwing up my sex life, if I was depressed about it or needed to talk. If I mentioned (as I was sobbing uncontrollably) that I wasn't doing too well, I could see the doctors physically tense up. They didn't want to talk. Whether it was because they didn't care or they felt bad because they couldn't do anything, I don't know. But surely, if someone comes into your office and you diagnose them with a rare condition for which there is no treatment, you should take their mental condition and quality of life into account. At least prescribe some antidepressants or Valium, for Christ's sake, if you can't be bothered to talk to them.

People with HS can be depressed or downright suicidal. They're often overweight, miss a lot of work, can't drive, exercise, or perform day-to-day tasks. They close themselves off from their friends and family, stay indoors away from people and isolate themselves. They're afraid that someone will find them out, perhaps that someone will smell the foul odor coming from their boils, or maybe even see one.

Or maybe they can't move without significant pain. Forget having sex. Besides being in excruciating pain, people with HS tend to think that no one would ever want to touch them.

I understand that some doctors may not be equipped emotionally to hold someone's hand through the pain, but attention needs to be paid to

SOPHIE'S STORY

I have had bumps and lumps for years and always assumed they were ingrown hairs. I finally realized (or maybe just accepted) that my lumps and bumps were a real problem. There have been so many times when I have just sat and cried to my husband saying:

"This is not fair!"

"Why do I have to live in agony?"

"This is NOT normal!"

When we finally realized I had HS, we were relieved to know that what I had was real. I had pointed out some bumps around my groin to my Ob-gyn. She told me it was a sebaceous cyst. Drink more water and use a warm compress. The advice seemed so trivial, like I am in pain all the time and your advice is to drink water ... I already drink more than enough!

So finally I knew what I had, and then I came to the sickening realization that there was nothing I could do about it. I wanted to curl up in a ball and cry. I mean here I am sitting, leaning to the right so as not to irritate the bump on my left "cheek," and propping my left arm up to alleviate the pain from my multiple bumps under my arm.

I read *The Paleo Diet* book months ago and had cut all the gluten I had been eating, but had not been too serious with dairy and had never even considered nightshades as being the culprit. Stumbling across this blog, I almost cried with relief (dramatic, I know, but I may be hypersensitive from current bump pain). I am just so thrilled that there could be the possibility of relief from painful bumps and lumps. I love potatoes, but I will throw those suckers away in a heartbeat if it means no more pain.

Sophie, no age given
United States

their patient's mental state. We need to know that someone understands.

We need education for doctors. The medical professionals I went to didn't even know what the condition was, let alone how to treat it. It took almost fifteen years to get a freakin' diagnosis. Part of this is our fault. People with HS don't talk about it. Doctors don't talk to each other about it. We don't share it with our friends or family.

We suffer in silence and shame.

That's why I wrote this book.

I wrote it because the modern Western medical system failed me and it is failing millions of you. Doctors are not equipped to give emotional support to HS patients, and psychiatrists are not equipped with the knowledge of how to stop the disease. There is no standardized treatment for HS. There is no real research, except to see how we react to different drugs or surgical procedures. We are being poked, prodded, cut, and medicated like guinea pigs.

We are being experimented on.

And we are being ignored.

I wrote this book because when I posted about HS on my website, thousands of you wrote me in need of help. Even though the posts have been up for over a year, hundreds of you continue to visit them every single day. Your stories are heartbreaking. I have included some of them here.

I wrote *Hidden Plague* because I have been HS-free for almost two years. Two entire years. I suffered from HS for over twenty years, with no more than two months in between flare-ups. Now, I am completely free of lesions, bumps, boils, zits, and ingrown hairs. Three years prior to complete remission, at the exact time I changed my diet, my HS retreated into mild stage I, with four- to five-month remission periods.

By doing extensive self-experimentation, I've been able to induce flare-ups—and to avoid them as well. I've also been able to reduce the healing time of a boil to less than twenty-four hours. I am in complete control of my HS, which, for some, might sound like an impossible goal.

This book is intended to help you identify what is actually causing your HS. There is way too much misinformation out there, some of which is downright dangerous. Once you truly understand what causes HS, you will be able to figure out what is causing it in *you*. In order to achieve this, we need to have a basic understanding of autoimmunity.

Understanding the connection between autoimmunity and leaky gut will help you understand why HS is the way it is, and why treatments like antibiotics and surgery don't work. Knowing what causes leaky gut and how to heal it will help you put your HS into remission.

Hidden Plague is organized into two sections: *The Whys and Wherefores of HS* and *The HS Autoimmune Protocol.* In the first section, you will learn the clinical definition of HS, how the medical community typically treats it, the root cause of HS (autoimmunity, caused by leaky gut), how stress and hormones can play a role, and how to care for your wounds.

The second section addresses the practical methods of kicking your HS into remission through diet. We'll discuss how to start an elimination diet to zero in on your personal food triggers. You'll receive detailed instructions on what to include in your self-designed paleo autoimmune diet—and what to avoid—and be introduced to some new and tasty recipes, including Tomato-Free Ketchup (page 210), to help you find substitutes for your favorite foods. I've also included a couple of sample journal pages from Mark Sisson's *Primal Blueprint 90-Day Journal* in the back of the book to get you started on tracking your progress.

I suggest that you first read this book in its entirety, before you try any experiments. If you skip ahead, you may miss a key piece of information, which could result in failure or frustration. Take notes along the way; perhaps you'll find something that you want to research in depth or something that is particularly pertinent to you.

This book is designed to help you identify most of the different factors that can cause an autoimmune response. That said, not everything mentioned in this guide is causing your HS. Everyone is different and autoimmune responses never seem to present the same way twice. So, if you try something that I've mentioned and it doesn't work, that could mean several things. (1) You may not have given it enough time, (2) you may be consuming a hidden trigger food, or—and sometimes this is really the answer—(3) that particular "tweak" just doesn't work for *you.* Just remember, the latest science on this topic backs me up. Really *try* it before you throw your hands up in defeat.

In order to be successful at this, you have to take charge of your health and your own destiny. You cannot approach this from a victim's perspective. Once you've read this book, you won't be able to use excuses anymore for why you have HS because you will have all the answers you need to get rid of it. I've kicked this thing's ass, and I am going to help you do the same.

For all of us afflicted, the time is here to come out of the closet. You now possess a name for the disease you have. You now know it's not contagious. You now have hope where there once was none. You now know it can get better.

I'm about to rock your world. Let's get going.

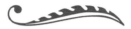

FOR FRIENDS & FAMILY

If you're a loved one of someone afflicted with this craptastic condition, there are a few things you should know:

You are an angel. Thank you for reading this. Having some insight into this disease can make all the difference in helping someone you love, since they probably won't tell you how much it's affecting them.

Your child/spouse/friend/lover needs you to understand that they are very embarrassed by this. Please don't point out new lesions unless you are asking about the disease directly or you're worried about infection. Trust me, they know they're there.

You will probably need to change your diet, especially if the person with HS is a child. The same foods that are affecting your kids are probably affecting you too. At the very least, it would be cruel to bust out the french fries at dinner and expect your kid to be OK with not having any. You may have to strong arm teenagers to change their eating habits, but they are usually quite motivated to look good, so perhaps not.

Your loved one needs to be touched and held, but they may be embarrassed or in pain when they are flaring up. A hug to let them know you're not afraid to touch them will really help.

Your loved one needs your discretion. Keep his or her condition to yourself. Don't go off talking about "Johnny's butt boil" at the next family reunion. Don't "out" them to anybody. They need to be able to trust you.

SJ'S STORY

I apologize for the sob story. Given that it's a pretty rare disease, I bet you are getting emails left and right on account of your article.

I really liked what you wrote and it seemed honest and not very doctor-ish. I am sick of hearing the same spiel from so many different doctors. When you're in pain, it's hard to sacrifice something that gives you pleasure, like food.

But, truthfully, I am trying this because I'm at the end of my rope. I wake up some mornings and wish I had died in my sleep. I cross the street and wish that a bus would hit me just so I wouldn't feel pain anymore. Constantly being told there's no cure has made me seriously consider killing myself. I am a very motivated, productive, hardworking guy ... so I want to try and work this out.

Can you give me some advice? You are the only person I have ever gotten in touch with who has HS, and I just want to know what your coping mechanisms were, what you started off doing with your diet, what exactly paleo is, how I should initiate this diet and how I should start eliminating different things.

I just want someone to talk to because I don't know anyone else who could possibly relate to me.

There's no support group that I know of for HS. I just need someone to give me some hope, some firsthand experience, just shine a light on this for me.

SJ, 25
Toronto, Canada

PART ONE:

THE WHYS AND WHEREFORES OF HS

CHAPTER ONE
What the Frak Is HS?

To diagnose hidradenitis, one first and foremost has to think of it.
—Jan von der Werth, dermatologist

Hidradenitis suppurativa is a debilitating chronic disease primarily affecting intertriginous skin of the axillae, perineum, and inframammary regions. The pathogenesis of this inflammatory disease is still poorly understood.

Oh wait, I'm sorry—you've probably already heard that from your doctor, who was reading it from a textbook. This account of HS was written by someone who doesn't have HS and who doesn't truly understand it. Words like "axillae" and "intertriginous" are thrown around like we're supposed to know what the hell they mean. Descriptions of HS are generally vague, short, and depressing, if you can understand them at all.

Please allow me to translate for you:

Hidradenitis suppurativa is a physically, psychologically, and socially disabling skin condition that shows up in the most sensitive parts of the human body: *inverse* areas—places where there is skin-to-skin contact. This means the armpits, under the breasts, the genitals, and the groin are all fair game. The disease manifests as incredibly painful boils, pus-filled abscesses, and hard lumps that can take months to heal, some-

Heat, stress, excess weight, hormonal changes, and excessive perspiration can all *worsen* the symptoms of HS, but none on their own actually *cause* HS.

times get infected, and most definitely leave scars. When the disease progresses, these sores often leak pus and can smell pretty bad. (This chronic seeping or leaking is known as *suppuration*, hence the name hidradenitis *suppurativa*.)

HS is recurrent, meaning sufferers flare-up over and over again, often one boil beginning to form before the last has had time to fully heal. According to HS-USA, an online support group, HS usually progresses from single boils filled with pus to painful, deep-seated, often inflamed clusters of lesions with significant scarring.[1]

HS is also known as *acne inversa*, or *Verneuil's disease*. Because flare-ups can occur near the genitals, they can resemble numerous sexually transmitted and contagious diseases. However, **HS is not contagious**. You didn't catch it from someone, and you can't give it to anyone either. The areas typically affected and the resemblance to a sexually transmitted disease is part of what makes HS so psychologically and socially damaging.

The medical community is stumped as to what causes HS, but they all seem to agree that it has something to do with inflammation ... or maybe sweat glands ... or perhaps obesity ... or maybe even polyester underwear. Scratch that, they don't have a clue. Very few doctors are able to recognize HS in the first place. When they do, the treatments they suggest are ineffective, temporary, and sometimes even harmful.[2]

If you are lucky enough to find a doctor who can actually diagnose you with HS, you will be told that there is neither a known cure, nor any consistently effective treatment for HS. You will be offered antibiotics, surgery, or both. You will not be offered hope, support, or anything that can actually help.

The Back(Side) Story

There is little to no awareness in the general public or the medical community about hidradenitis suppurativa. Considering it was first diagnosed in 1839, you'd think more people would have heard about it by now. Most doctors don't learn about it in medical school—they get their first taste of HS when a teary, boil-ridden patient shows up in their office demanding a cure.

Over the last 170 years, there has been exactly no progress in the treatment or cure of HS.[3] "Is this so?" writes expert dermatologist Jan von der Werth in his 2000 article "The natural history of hidradenitis suppurativa," published in *Dermatology in Practice*, a review-based journal dedicated to dermatology. "Have we really failed to advance significantly on this disease despite our powerful array of modern medicaments and surgical techniques? I guess in the eyes of many who suffer from HS the answer would be: yes. Hands up all those who feel comfortable when confronted with a hidradenitis patient."[4]

No doubt about it, doctors are stumped and do *not* feel comfortable when we visit them with our boils. They just don't know what to do for us.

There have been several problems that have set us back in our quest to find answers. First and foremost, there have been major misunderstandings about what actually causes HS. The misguided belief that HS was a disease of the sweat, or *apocrine*, glands became quickly accepted by the medical community and many people received treatments for presumed apocrine gland infections, with no benefit at all.[5]

It wasn't until the 1990s that a series of detailed studies on HS were conducted. The studies found that sweat glands

TELLTALE SIGNS OF HS

Blackheads: small, pitted areas of skin containing blackheads, sometimes appearing in pairs.

Tender lumps and bumps: Very often, these bumps will get bigger, break open, and drain pus. They turn red, itch, burn, and may have an unpleasant odor. Sometimes they vanish mysteriously without getting bigger or draining.

Painful pea-sized lumps: These hard lumps develop underneath the skin and may persist for years. Sometimes they get bigger and become inflamed.

Leaking bumps and sores: Open wounds which heal slowly, if at all. They often lead to scarring and the development of sinus tracts (i.e., tunnels) under the skin.[17]

These lumps, bumps, boils, tunnels, and blackheads can appear anywhere on the body, but are most often found in places where skin touches skin: the groin, the armpits, under the breasts, the genital area, and the buttocks.

Some people only have one area of their body affected. Others have symptoms in multiple regions. Sometimes, symptoms will disappear from one area and reappear in another.

People with HS can also suffer from scalp nodules, cystic acne, and pilondial cysts. Please see "Follicular Occlusion" on page 22 for more information.

only become involved when there is intense inflammation,[6] and are actually not the cause of the disease. Despite this knowledge, removal of the sweat glands is still suggested and carried out in severe cases. This drastic procedure has yet to be proven effective. The study concluded that HS is primarily an acne-like disease where the hair follicles become blocked, resulting in the inflammatory skin condition.

Unfortunately your doctor hears "acne-like" and thinks that standard acne treatments should be effective. They are not. HS is not acne. Yet, doctors continue to prescribe these courses of treatment because they don't know what else to do to get you out of their office.

Another part of the problem is that researchers, doctors, and even patients themselves draw conclusions about HS based on correlation, i.e., coincidence. HS has been linked to other conditions such as diabetes and PCOS, but not all HS sufferers have diabetes or PCOS. Some studies have linked it to cigarette smoking,[7] but not everyone with HS smokes. Medical studies have made a connection between HS and obesity,[8] HS and Crohn's disease, HS and ulcerative colitis, HS and IBD,[9] and HS and tight pants. There is incredible misinformation out there. Everyone seems to present their symptoms slightly differently. No one seems to have just HS. It's always HS and ... acne. Or IBS. Or Hashimoto's. Or eczema, depression, endometriosis, or arthritis. Shall I continue? It's not surprising so many of us smoke.[10] (We'll explore the correlation between HS and tobacco in chapter eight, *Phase I: The Elimination Diet.*)

On some level, the very people who suffer from HS bear some responsibility for the lack of medical advancement in this matter. "Any researcher in the field will confirm the reluctance of patients with [HS] to come forward with their disease," writes Dr. von der Werth. "Patients frequently conceal their condition even from their closest relatives.... The patient's evasiveness coupled with the lack of diagnostic laboratory tests have probably led to significant underreporting of HS, betraying its true significance and condemning it to a fringe existence among over one thousand other dermatological conditions."[11]

Estimates indicate that anywhere from one to twelve million people have HS in the United States alone.[12] To put that into perspective, that means there are more HS sufferers in the US than those living with HIV or AIDS.[13] This isn't an American problem; HS doesn't discriminate. It's worldwide and is reaching epidemic proportions.

Enter the Internet

If you've had HS for longer than ten years, I know there was once a time when you thought you were the only person in the world with it. Even your doctor didn't know what was wrong with you. I sure know I felt isolated and afraid to open up.

Today is different. Information, stories, and images of HS are everywhere online, as more people "come out" anonymously. There are forums, websites, and Facebook groups dedicated to the disease. Some are nothing other than places where people can vent, ask questions, and connect. We finally have an online presence, and we know we're not alone.

The problem is, we're united online but no one has any answers. No one seems to know why the HS sometimes gets worse, or why it migrates to different places on the body. No one really knows what causes it in the first place. Everyone is desperate and grasping at straws, trying anything they've heard will work to end the pain.

Just like you, I started looking for any information I could find online about my condition. I searched and searched and came up pretty much empty-handed.

I found stupid—just bloody *stupid*—treatments online, from the hacks trolling Yahoo Answers, to the standard literature about how there is no cure, there will never *be* a cure, and "This is your cross to bear; get used to it." Of course, there were also horror stories about HS surgery—complete with new boils popping up through newly graphed skin and stitches, causing unbearable agony and horrific scarring. Most of the sufferers were either on some sort of antibiotic (or had been in the near past), were contemplating surgery, or even thinking about killing themselves. From what I could tell from the online image search, I considered myself lucky as hell. Some people were suffering so badly that I broke down and cried.

On average, HS begins around twenty-three years of age. It affects women two to five times more often than men. In severe cases, boils can erupt in any hair-bearing part of the body.

The forums were not a good place for me. I do not take comfort in collective suffering. I want answers, solutions, and effective treatments.

If you don't have this condition, thank whatever gods you pray to. Then take a look around: I bet you know at least five—if not more—people with this disease. There was a time when I was the only person I knew willing to start a conversation about it. But once I opened up to a couple of friends, they had a lot to say. They told me that they had it too—they just didn't know what it was called, what was causing it, or how to get rid of it.

I've gotten pretty good at spotting HS, and have seen signs of it on more than one occasion. I recently tuned into NBC's *The Biggest Loser* and saw three different contestants with signs of HS in their armpits. If you still feel alone and isolated, just open your eyes. This condition is rampant.

FOLLICULAR OCCLUSION SYNDROME (FOS)

If you've got HS in the standard regions, chances are you have problems with the skin on other parts of your body too. You may have facial acne, ingrown hairs in your nose, zits on your scalp, chicken skin on your upper arms, calluses that grow excessively on the bottom of your feet, something besides the boils on your butt.

Follicular occlusion syndrome (FOS) refers to a group of four diseases in which hair follicles become blocked with keratin (scale) and then rupture—resulting in the pain and inflammation we've all come to know and love. FOS covers hidradenitis suppurativa (of course), plus acne conglobata (HS on your face), dissecting cellulitis (HS on your scalp), and pilonidal disease (HS around your tailbone). Although keratin is also responsible for regular acne, hyperkeratosis pillaris (chicken skin), and zits in your nose, somehow those conditions didn't make it into the FOS tetrad club.

Doctors realized that all these conditions commonly coexist, that they are very similar, and they are all difficult to treat, but they didn't know why. So, they went ahead and created a disease for each area of the body that was affected, grouped them altogether in a "syndrome," and haven't found an effective treatment for any of them since. The "diseases" of FOS are actually all the same disease (autoimmunity), attacking the same thing (the hair follicle), but just in different areas of the body. They are all caused by the same things—and fixed by the same things—as HS.

Since you have HS, you can readily assume that your body's keratin making mechanism is off—since keratin plays a role in FOS diseases. To find out what you can do to get it working properly again, read up on vitamin A on page 89.

The Stages of HS

HURLEY STAGE	EXTENT OF DISEASE IN TISSUE
I	Abscess formation (single or multiple) without sinus tracts and cicatrization
II	One or more widely separated recurrent abscesses with tract formation and scars
III	Multiple interconnected tracts and abscesses throughout an entire area

There are different stages to HS. It can be progressive and aggressive. In some, the disease progresses relentlessly. Others may only experience mild symptoms their entire lives. One system physicians refer to is called Hurley's Staging,[14] yet few apparently have actually studied (or understand) it, as they should be able to tell patients what to expect if they had.

To the layperson, the Hurley's Staging system is filled with hard-to-understand medical terms and brief descriptions so vague that a lot of people are confused as to how the disease progresses, exactly what to expect, and when to be scared. It doesn't provide treatment options, either. The system is simply a diagnostic tool.

The lines between the different stages of HS can certainly be blurred; you may have stage I HS in your armpits while suffering from stage II or even III in your groin. One thing is for certain: all the stages suck.

With stage I and II, the disease tends to affect the hair follicles. In stage III, it affects the sweat glands. This is serious stuff. Boils will cluster and concentrate in areas where your sweat glands are: mainly your groin and armpits. Instead of the lackadaisical pattern of stage I and II, where you can see some skin between the abscesses, in this stage, there's no skin left.

Regardless of whether it's oversimplified, misleading, hard to understand, or just plain wrong, Hurley's Staging system is pretty much all we have to go on at the moment. I'll do my best to translate it for you on the following pages.

Stage I

Stage I HS is mild compared to the other stages. Some sufferers may not even know they have it. Strange painful lumps, zits, and boils appear from time to time—just once or twice a year in some cases—and disappear. There might be one lump, there may be two or three. They're small most of the time. Some people think they just have acne on their bums or ingrown hairs in their armpits. HS will often start off as a single, painful lump that persists for weeks or months, and then simply goes away.

Breakouts can be on the groin, buttocks, pubic area, upper thighs, in the armpit, or on or under the breasts. They can even be on the penis and testicles for men.

A person might experience a flare-up so mild it could be mistaken for acne, and later experience a rare, super painful boil with lots of inflammation, swelling, and drainage. It's not uncommon for people in stage I to also experience similar episodes of acne on their face, neck, and other places.

Since it doesn't pose much of a problem (except for embarrassment), stage I sufferers tend to not seek help, get a diagnosis, or tell anyone about it. They may not know what they have, much less how to treat it. They may use standard acne treatments with some success or notice that flare-ups get worse from time to time.

In stage I HS, flare-ups tend to be singular and small. In stage II, those boils get sick of the single life and join together for a friendly meet and greet.

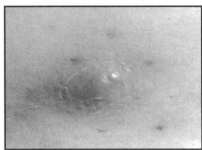

STAGE I

A single boil, surrounded by small scars.

Credit: Tanya Newiadomy. Used with permission.

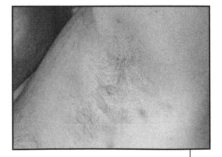

STAGE I

Some breakouts are so mild they may be mistaken for acne.

Credit: BMC Dermatology. Used with permission.

Stage II

You really start to notice HS when you reach stage II. The painful lumps become bigger and can turn into large boils, which erupt after an excruciatingly long time (sometimes weeks). Pus comes out, just like a pimple, but so does blood. Once erupted, these boils can *suppurate* (or leak and ooze) for ages. They can take weeks to come to a head and sometimes take months to heal. Many people in stage II have at least two boils on their body, in varying degrees of healing. The lucky ones are granted a reprieve for a month or two.

Some patients go to the doctor to have a stage II boil lanced, but find that the lesion never fully heals.[15] In fact, it's fairly common for another boil to pop up in the same place before the previous one has fully healed. Also common in stage II are hard, deep-seated, extremely painful lumps. These lumps are particularly frustrating because they never come to the surface of the skin and resolve.

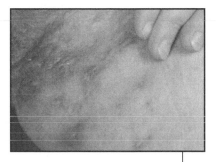

STAGE II

Sinus tracts create their own special kind of scars.

Credit: BMC Dermatology. Used with permission.

Scarring in stage II also becomes significant. Clusters of boils may appear and take several months to resolve while others come and go on different parts of the body. Boils may tunnel under the skin and leave twisted *sinus tract* scars along the infected area. Doctors will almost invariably suggest incision and drainage at this stage, and you have a super big chance of infection if you're not careful. When stage II worsens, you may start missing work, bowing out of social (or intimate) situations, or have your movement restricted in some way.

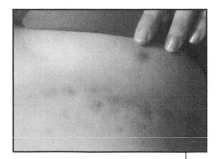

STAGE II

Scarring becomes significant.

Credit: Danielle Harker. Used with permission.

Stage III

In stage III, the boils can become as big as a golf ball—sometimes the size of baseballs, although this is rare. The lesions often join together, become bigger, and form protruding clusters, not unlike the way bath bubbles cluster together to form larger bubbles.

The pain that occurs in stage III is overwhelming, and patients are typically unable to function. When it's this bad, HS affects every area of your life, restricts your movement, and impacts your state of mind. It's gone way past being an embarrassment. It has officially become a debilitating disease.

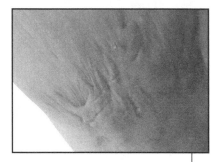

STAGE II-III
Sinus Tracts create their own type of scarring.
Credit: Danielle Harker. Used with permission

HS attacks the sweat glands when there is intense inflammation going on in the body. If you're in stage III, the other symptoms you may experience include horrible headaches, cramps, joint pain, and depression.

People in stage III are usually the ones who finally resort to surgery. They've exhausted all the options their doctors offer without success and are left only with risky medications or procedures. Sometimes, healing from the invasive surgery can be less painful than dealing with the HS. I've been told the surgical scars are easier to bear than the scars caused by the boils.

It will take longer for people in stage III to heal than it will for someone whose symptoms are mild, but it can be done. Don't give up hope.

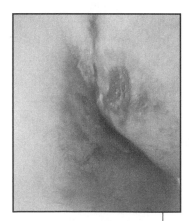

STAGE III
Scarring and
Active Infection
Credit: Kiley MacLeod. Used with permission

It Does Get Better

It's a common misconception that HS progresses like cancer. Perhaps it's because Hurley's Staging System uses the term "stages." Frightened HS patients immediately associate this with cancer when they are told they are "in stage IV, diagnosis terminal. Treatment options exhausted. Prepare to die."

HS is nothing like cancer. You don't get stage I and relentlessly deteriorate until you reach stage III and are confined to a hospital bed, frantically writing your last will and testament. Some people present immediately in stage III while others present in stage I, move to stage II, regress back to stage I and so on—but they never reach stage III. At the same time, going to the doctor for the first time and being placed in stage III doesn't mean that you've ignored the problem or let it go too long. **HS doesn't always relentlessly progress.**[16]

If the doctor tells you that you have a specific stage of HS, it is simply a way of diagnosing how bad the disease is at the present time. There is nothing saying that you are going to get worse. In fact, if you make some changes to your diet and your lifestyle, your HS will get better. No chemotherapy required.

WHY YOU SHOULD GO TO THE DOCTOR

If you haven't been diagnosed, you first need to make sure that what you have is actually HS. Second, you need to make sure that you don't have any life-threatening infections. Third, if you do have HS, there needs to be a record of it.

Most HS sufferers don't go to the doctor so the statistics are off—way off. According to HS-USA, there are one million people in the US diagnosed with HS, but they estimate it's more like twelve million.[1] I personally think it's even higher than that, but twelve million is pretty substantial by itself. The only way we can truly raise awareness of this disease is to come out of the closet.

Before You Go

Make sure you've read this book and researched the disease. You will be armed with tools to make decisions about your medical future. Will you take the antibiotics the doctor inevitably prescribes? Will you opt for surgery? Or leave with just a diagnosis and the knowledge that you are going to heal yourself? The power is in your hands.

Once You're Diagnosed

First off, don't panic. If you're suffering from stage I or stage II HS, you're not necessarily going to careen into stage III. Even if you do nothing, you may never progress beyond the stage you are in currently. The point is, getting diagnosed with HS is not a death sentence. Even if you are already in stage III, there is hope that you can get better. Everyone is different and each case of HS is unique, which is why HS is sometimes hard to diagnose. Read through the rest of this book to find a plan that works best for you.

CHAPTER TWO
What the Doctors Will Tell You

> *Each patient carries his own doctor inside him.*
> —Norman Cousins, *Anatomy of an Illness*

e've established that the medical community is some-what clueless when it comes to HS. They don't know what causes it, how to treat it, or what our long-term prognosis is. They don't understand the emotional turmoil, the excruciating pain, or the shame we feel.

If you go to the doctor's office with a really bad flare-up or to discuss treatment options, you will more than likely be presented with the options listed in this chapter. If you are in excruciating pain, you may want a quick and easy way out. If you're tired of dealing with flare-ups that seemingly occur for no reason, you may be tempted to try something new. Although pharmaceutical interventions may seem to be the easiest solution at the time, please be advised that any treatment options your doctor may provide could have mild benefits now—and dire consequences later.

This chapter discusses theories and treatments you may encounter at the doctor's office so that you may make informed decisions for yourself—decisions based on *science*—as opposed to misinformation. Remember, your doctor probably doesn't know what causes HS or how to effectively treat your symptoms. Doctors are still using outdated, incorrect information and treatments that have been shown to be ineffective. Most of them are still unaware of the fact that HS is an autoimmune condition.

They'll Tell You It's Hygiene

"YOU NEED TO KEEP EXTRA CLEAN"

For some reason unknown to scientific logic and reason, many doctors still believe that bacteria cause HS. Even after science has ruled out MRSA, staph, or any number of super bugs, the medical community continues to maintain this unfounded idea. This is probably because for the last 150 years, the traditional medical community's approach to disease has been based on the germ theory. The theory states that disease is caused by exposure to pathogenic organisms from the environment.[2] There is absolutely no attention paid to what is going on inside the body.

So doctors prescribe antibiotics to deal with perceived bacteria. They recommend antibacterial soaps and washes to use on your skin. They tell you that you need to keep extra clean and wash more.

This makes us feel dirty and ashamed. Because, as much as we scrub and as many antibiotics we take, the HS keeps coming back. We must be doing *something* wrong.

Maybe you shower or bathe daily, use antibacterial washes, scrub at the boils, and frantically wash the parts of your body where boils like to pop up until they're raw. You hit the showers the second your workout is over, rinsing away any sweat and all those horrible, horrible bacteria with it. You bathe in chlorine to kill any germs that may be present. This isn't your fault. You've been told that this will help. You've been made to feel ashamed of your hygiene and your habits.

Again, HS is not a bacterial infection. Washing three times a day is not going to make it go away—in fact, it may even make it worse!

> I felt entirely invisible and uncomfortably obvious all at the same time, sitting there in practically nothing in front of this stranger who was ignoring me.
>
> —Jessica Verdi,
> *My Life After Now*

Unfortunately old habits die hard. If you've been doing this for years, you may still feel compelled to keep fastidiously clean.

I agree that people with HS need to pay attention to sensitive areas where hair grows, like the pubic area and underarms. And yes, we need to keep our lesions clean and free from infection. I'm not saying you can stop taking showers for weeks on end—no one wants to be the smelly kid. What I'm talking about here is OCD washing. You shouldn't be ritually scrubbing your skin everyday or soaking in bleach. It's just not good for you. Not only are you hurting your skin, you're hurting the delicate balance of your skin flora.

HS flare-ups are the result of something going wrong inside the body; you can't prevent them from outside—no matter how much you scrub. Give your skin a break. It bears the brunt of this disease. It isn't the cause.

"IT'S CAUSED BY SWEATING"

Once upon a time, HS was thought to be a disease of the apocrine (sweat) glands. This theory was first raised in the 1800s, and was scientifically debunked in the early 1990s. Stage III HS does affect the sweat glands, but your sweat glands don't cause HS. Neither does sweating.

The fact that doctors in the twenty-first century would suggest using antiperspirant, Botox, or even the surgical removal of all your sweat glands to help slow the progress of HS goes to show you that they're grasping at straws.

As far as I can figure out, the theory goes something like this: most people with HS have a problem with their weight. Overweight people sweat more than thinner people. HS can affect the sweat glands. Therefore, sweating causes HS.

Blaming sweat for HS makes about as much sense as blaming vomit—a side effect of excess alcohol—for cirrhosis of the liver.

Even though the treatment is based on decades-old faulty information, sweat gland removal surgery is still often suggested for HS patients. A quick google search turned up testimonials of people who had tried the surgery. Here's one:

I had surgery for sweat gland removal years ago. It kept HS away for about four years, and it returned, but not as bad as before at first. It's been ten years now, and flares are becoming more frequent. —Karen at MdJunction.com

If you suffer from HS and have also noticed that you sweat excessively, you may have a hormonal imbalance. As we'll learn in chapter five, *The Hormone Connection*, our hormones are interconnected and strive to achieve balance within our bodies. If you have low levels of the hormone *aldosterone*, your sodium excretion mechanism can get thrown out of whack, consequently resulting in excess sweating. Cutting down on dietary sodium and reducing stress will go much further towards fixing this problem than covering it up with antiperspirant or removing your sweat glands.

"YOU SHOULD WEAR COTTON UNDERWEAR AND LOOSE FITTING CLOTHES"

This was the first advice I was ever given by a doctor regarding HS. At the time it made sense. Cotton allows your skin to breathe and loose fitting clothes are much more comfortable than tight ones, especially tight clothes that rub against a flare-up. As the years progressed, I alternated between heeding this advice and forgetting about it completely. Over time, I realized that it didn't seem to matter whether I followed it or not.

Some people with HS notice that heat and humidity affect their flare-ups. If this applies to you, you will probably want to choose loose-fitting clothing made of cotton so that your skin can breathe, moisture isn't trapped, and you aren't in pain. Just remember that polyester doesn't cause HS. These recommendations are simply for comfort.

They'll Recommend Medications

Let's be clear about something right off the bat: **there are no drugs out there that will cure your HS.** Here, we'll look at specific medications you're likely to encounter at the doctor's office. Understand that none of these will *cure* your HS. Some of them will actually make it worse.

Keep in mind that some doctors are starting to get frighteningly creative, since nothing they've prescribed in the past seems to work. You may very well be prescribed a new drug with a different name that is usually given to patients with diseases different from yours. As the medical community becomes more desperate to find a pharmacological cure or treatment for HS, you will continue to have the honor of being treated like a guinea pig to see what works—and what doesn't.

It is completely up to you whether or not you try medication. If your doctor feels like experimenting (and you feel like being experimented on), make sure that your doctor at least tries a drug that has been shown to have an effect on other autoimmune issues. Although these medications may seem to have some positive short-term effects on HS, please be advised that some—like TNFα blockers—can cause terrible long-term problems, including cancer, seizure, and death.

Something else to consider: patients who have been prescribed these heavy-hitting drugs often can't tolerate them for long. Any relief from HS is completely reversed when medication is stopped, and, as a consequence of taking such strong medication, many are often left with a brand new illness to contend with.

"YOU NEED TO TAKE ANTIBIOTICS"

The medication traditionally dispensed for HS is antibiotics. By its very definition, antibiotics "inhibit the growth of, or destroy, microorganisms."[3] This is absolutely wonderful if you are plagued with a bacterial, parasitic, or fungal infection. Problem is, HS isn't caused by any of those things. Taking antibiotics will not get rid of HS and in time will likely make it even worse.

Once you read chapters three and four, and know the true cause of HS, you'll understand why taking antibiotics for this condition is such an absurd idea. It's so absurd, in fact, that I would go so far as to say that prescribing antibiotics for HS is negligent.

Bacteria, including the good guys in our guts, are microorganisms. It isn't even controversial to say that antibiotics decimate our gut flora. And when that happens, our guts repopulate with bad microorganisms because much of the good bacteria has been killed off. This is what is known of as *dysbiosis,* an imbalance in the ratio of beneficial to harmful bacteria in our gut.

Some of the side effects I experienced from compromised gut flora due to antibiotics included recurrent yeast infections, recurrent strep throat, recurrent tonsillitis, frequent colds, fatigue, IBS, and depression. And, of course,

> *Most therapies used to treat HS are supported by limited or weak scientific evidence.*
>
> —Archives of Dermatology, 2012

there was always the antibiotic-associated diarrhea. Ever wonder what that is?

Well, some bad bacteria are resistant to antibiotics, and this number is growing by the day with increased use of the drugs. Normally, the beneficial bacteria in our guts keep harmful, antibiotic-resistant bacteria, like *Clostridium difficile*, in check. But without the good bacteria around to soldier up, the antibiotic-resistant bad guys grow out of control and produce toxins that damage the gut wall, trigger inflammation, and kick-start autoimmune responses. This affects the way that we metabolize foods and liquids and ultimately results in diarrhea.

And then there's the antibiotic-associated constipation. Poor gut flora is the number one cause of constipation. When you're constipated, lipo-polysaccharide (LPS) toxins and other endotoxins that would normally just keep moving and get cleared out of the intestines get stuck instead. When toxins hang around too long, they damage the gut lining and make it permeable.[4] This opens the door for autoimmunity, digestive disorders, and all sorts of other problems.

That's why no matter what I took antibiotics for, or for how long I took them, my HS was always there. The lowered immunity, diarrhea, and constipation I experienced due to taking antibiotics actually made my HS worse in the long run.

Your doctor is supposed to check for signs of infection before administering antibiotics, but a lot of them don't. If your doctor *confirms* an infection, a short course of *systemic antibiotics,* such as clindamycin, or a *macrolide antibiotic,* like clarithromycin, are the most effective for HS-related infection.[5] Keep in mind, these drugs will only help with the current infection—they won't actually make your HS go away.

Some doctors prescribe short courses of penicillin or some other antibiotic. This is actually a frequent mistake. These drugs are not effective for the treatment of HS—as virtually every HS patient already knows.[6]

Medical research conducted in the year 2000 found that any benefit antibiotics seem to have is coincidental. "It seems striking that the mean duration of an HS boil (6.9 days) roughly equals the duration of an average course of antibiotics," writes Dr. Van der Werth. "The postulated response of HS to oral antibiotics may thus simply have its explanation in the natural history of the condition itself."[7]

Doctors who still believe bacteria cause HS will often prescribe longer courses of antibiotics. Because of the cyclical nature of HS, they may believe that keeping the antibiotics in your system for months, or even *years*, will eventually kill off the bacteria that are causing it. Since we now know that HS is an autoimmune condition—and not a bacterial infection—this line of treatment no longer makes sense.

Antibiotics should be saved for life-threatening infections. If you have to take them, supplement with a beneficial yeast like *Saccharomyces boulardii* (brand name *Florastor*). This yeast has been proven to prevent diarrhea associated with antibiotics,[8] and has even been shown to be more effective on its own than antibiotics for some parasitic infections.[9] After you have finished a course of antibiotics, you should follow it up with a course of regular probiotics to help repopulate and heal your intestines.

Even if it's been years since you've last had antibiotics, you're likely still suffering from dysbiosis. Supplementing with quality probiotics needs to be part of your routine if you hope to put your HS into remission. Fermented foods are also great for populating the gut with beneficial bacteria, but they contain yeast by-products, which can be problematic for many of us. We'll discuss gut dysbiosis, probiotics, and yeast as a trigger as we progress further into other chapters.

Just know that for now, if you have taken antibiotics quite a few times in your life, the effects can last for years—the damage a lifetime, if you don't do something about it. Save the antibiotics for when you've contracted a bacterial infection for which there is no other treatment.

WHAT ARE CYTOKINES?

Cytokines are chemical messengers in our blood that are made by immune cells. It's their job to tell white blood cells—our immune system's warriors—to attack. Everyone has cytokines—they're a super important part of the immune system. High levels of cytokines in your blood, organs, or tissue means your body thinks it's under attack and is launching an immune response. Patients with autoimmune disorders have high levels of inflammatory cytokines in affected tissue.

Inflammatory cytokines can trigger the release of even more cytokines and usually result in chronic inflammation and other immune responses. HS lesions and HS-affected skin have been shown to contain high levels of inflammatory cytokines.[17] This is scientific proof that HS is an autoimmune response.

MORE ON ANTIBIOTICS

Some people who are prescribed antibiotics for their HS sometimes go into a period of remission at first. I have heard story after story expressing a similar sentiment: "The antibiotics just stopped working after several months." I have a personal theory about this.

In 2011, I was hospitalized for severe abdominal pain, the cause of which was never discovered. Initial blood tests showed I had an elevated white blood cell (WBC) count so without my permission, I was given mega-doses of intravenous antibiotics. Turns out, I didn't actually have an active infection; the doctors ran every test under the sun and couldn't find a thing wrong with me—except for the elevated WBCs. Immediately upon administration of the antibiotics, my WBC count started to decrease, which the doctors took as a good sign. But it didn't stop decreasing.

After two days, I had a WBC count less than that of a chemotherapy patient. The hospital staff had to wear masks around me, sterilize my room, and I wasn't allowed to leave the hospital for five days. I was labeled leucopenic, meaning that I had an abnormally low number of WBCs. Any exposure to infection or germs could have taken me out.

At the time, I knew that antibiotics decimated your gut flora, but I didn't know that they had the capacity to wipe out your white blood cells too. This doesn't normally happen, according to medical literature. I couldn't find a single study on it. Antibiotics are supposed to work together with white blood cells to destroy bacteria. As soon as I was taken off of the antibiotics, my WBC count started to slowly increase. It took about a month for it to return to normal levels. So what happened?

Dr. Tim Gerstmar, a naturopathic doctor at Asprire Natural Health, a Washington-based natural healing clinic, was able to uncover some information. Although what he found was "spotty," he did discover that a good number of antibiotics can cause low WBC counts in up to 7 percent of patients, after taking the drugs five or more days. He also found that it can take anywhere from three to thirty days to recover. "So, it can happen, but it's not really common and tends to happen with extended use of antibiotics," he writes. "But more interesting to me was I could not find, despite some serious searching, any explanation of how any of the antibiotics cause this to happen."[10]

Perhaps this phenomenon is more common than we think, especially with those suffering from autoimmune issues. How many times in your life have you been prescribed antibiotics? And how many times has your doctor done follow-up blood tests to see what your WBC count is? My answers are: (1) too many times to count (at least thirty) and (2) once—while I was in the hospital and hooked up to an IV. Otherwise, I have never had a doctor perform a blood test after I have taken antibiotics. If my symptoms are gone, it is assumed I am "good to go." I have, however, always experienced some sort of illness or serious infection after taking antibiotics.

Most HS patients have higher than normal amounts of inflammatory cytokines circulating in their blood. Every cell in your immune system produces cytokines, including a type of lymphocyte called T-helper cells. T-helper cells are a type of white blood cell. Cytokines are produced when the T-helper cell recognizes a foreign invader.[11] Simply put, cytokines are messengers that carry a message from one cell to another, potentially anywhere in your body, and help to regulate the immune response. Another role they play is in stimulating the production of more T-helper cells. This can result in an endless feedback loop[12] and in theory, a high WBC count.

It is my theory that, along with elevated cytokine levels, WBC counts in general are probably higher in HS patients than in the average person. I have spoken to several women afflicted with HS who have confirmed that they, too, have high WBC counts. If someone takes antibiotics, which in turn destroy some of their WBCs, there are fewer WBCs to launch the initial attack. It makes sense that this could result in HS flare-ups that are either less frequent, less violent, or that even disappear for a while. We don't know how this happens but antibiotic treatment has been shown to be effective enough— short term anyway—to become a popular treatment for HS over the last few decades, so it is happening somehow.

This could explain why extended antibiotic use in some HS patients may be effective for a period of time. However, since we now know that HS is an autoimmune response (not a bacterial infection) it makes absolutely no sense to take antibiotics for it—especially since the long-term effects of antibiotics are worse than any short-term benefits you may have.

DANIELLE'S STORY

In 2006 I was diagnosed with hidradenitis and was given antibiotics, creams, lotions, and potions but nothing ever worked. All they did was give me irritable bowel syndrome, but I kept on at my doctor and in 2008 I was given surgery under my arms. I had a terrible time. I even caught MRSA from the hospital I had surgery at. After I'd healed up, which took me about eight months due to the MRSA, I thought I was in the clear and surgery had worked but I woke up one morning with an abscess on my inner thigh, which quickly spread causing it to track along the leg. It has now left me with ten lesions, which leak and bleed out of about thirteen holes. It has spread into my "lady garden" recently, and it has spread to my bottom. Over the years, I thought of suicide as a way out, but I couldn't leave my children. I have had mental breakdowns, serious bouts of depression because I just want to be normal if there is such a thing.

I won't have any more surgery because of how vicious the HS came back after the arm operation, so I'm at a loss now. I've tried all sorts of medicine, I've tried manuka honey, giving up smoking, weight loss, all kinds of diets. It just doesn't want to leave me and my body alone.

Danielle, 30
Kent, United Kingdom

"ACNE MEDICATION MIGHT HELP"

Let's face it—acne medication rarely works, even on regular acne. Because of the similarities between HS and cystic acne, doctors often prescribe acne medications to treat the condition.

Acne medications—including Accutane, Retinol, and Proactiv—do not help prevent HS. They can irritate and thin out the skin, cause redness and flaking, and make conditions even more painful. Furthermore, Accutane was recalled in 2009 due to serious side effects, including inflammatory bowel disease, liver damage, depression, miscarriage, and birth defects. Generic versions of Accutane known as *isotretinoin* are, however, still available and are widely prescribed. A dermatologist offered me a prescription for isotretinoin for mild HS symptoms in 2010. I politely declined.

Over-the-counter topical acne solutions like salicylic acid and benzoyl peroxide aren't effective for HS either, although they aren't as harmful as some other options. I have used both of these solutions on lesions over the years, and while they did nothing to aid healing, stop the process, or prevent new boils, the boils I already had didn't get infected. Furthermore, salicylic acid is beneficial for exfoliating. Rubbing alcohol, although painful, is particularly good at drying out a wound, preventing infection, and is much cheaper than acne medication.

Although I personally hate it when doctors treat HS like it's acne, I have to admit that there are many things that a pimple and a boil have in common. In fact, the formation and growth process of both pimples and boils are almost identical. Anything that has been *clinically proven* to cause acne will invariably cause problems with HS as well. That said, a topical approach simply does not address the underlying problem. It is more appropriate to apply standard wound care and treat the lesions like what they really are—boils—instead of treating HS like acne. I really wish doctors would stop treating HS like it's a case of teenage zits.

For more information on how to care for a flare-up, please read chapter six, *Wound Care*.

"TAKE NON-STEROIDAL ANTI-INFLAMMATORY DRUGS"

NSAIDs such as aspirin, ibuprofen, and naproxen, work by blocking prostaglandins. Prostaglandins are hormone-like substances that circulate throughout the body, signaling pain and promoting healing. When you take NSAIDs, you may temporarily alleviate the pain, but you also block the healing process.[13] The problem you're trying to treat doesn't go away just because you managed to block the pain. In fact, the problem sticks around much longer than it would have otherwise. And that's not all.

NSAIDs also affect the digestive tract, which repairs and replaces itself about every three days. NSAIDs block that repair, and if overused will eventually cause the lining of the intestines to become inflamed, putting you at a higher risk for leaky gut.

"LET'S PUT YOU ON CORTICOSTEROIDS"

According to Dr. von der Werth, the quickest way for relief of an acute painful boil is systemic corticosteroids. Examples of this type of drug include hydrocortisone and prednisone. These compounds limit certain parts of the immune response and reduce inflammation. Von der Werth recommends 30 mg of prednisone for three or four days.[14]Prednisone is one of the most widely used systemic steroids. It has amazing anti-inflammatory effects. In addition to oral dosage form, it is available for subcutaneous, intramuscular, and intravenous injection.[15] Prednisone is also prescribed for other autoimmune conditions, such as multiple sclerosis.

Caution should be used if you resort to corticosteroids. While they can reduce the pain and inflammation of a flare-up, they won't prevent new ones—in fact, corticosteroids are a proven cause of leaky gut, so although they will relieve immediate pain, they can actually delay healing and cause more problems down the road. One person I spoke to actually developed HS after taking prednisone for an unrelated matter —and she only flares when she takes the medication.

If you do take corticosteroids, don't take them for long periods of time as they have multiple long-term side effects, including adrenal gland suppression, immune suppression, and protein breakdown.[16] If you are pregnant, you can't take prednisone. If you are female and of childbearing age, your doctor should ask you a billion questions and make you sign a waiver before taking it. This is big league stuff, baby.

"LET'S REDUCE THE INFLAMMATION WITH TNFA BLOCKERS"

Pro-inflammatory cytokines are important in the immune response to infections and, although they are present in all humans, they are found in higher-than-normal levels in autoimmune patients. Elevated cytokines, in particular interleukin (IL)-1β and tumor necrosis factor alpha (TNFα)[18]—in HS patients is evidence that HS is autoimmune in nature.

TNFα causes the inflammatory process that is associated with many autoimmune disorders, including rheumatoid arthritis, inflammatory bowel disease, psoriasis, and asthma. Large amounts can mess up insulin signaling and create insulin resistance. If that weren't enough, TNFα also stimulates the interaction among the hypothalamus, pituitary, and adrenal glands—appropriately known as the hypothalamus-pituitary-adrenal (HPA) axis—to release large amounts of *corticotropin-releasing hormone* (CRH), which in turn can cause depression and hypoglycemia. (See page 251 for more information on CRH.) Large amounts of TNFα are released in response to LPS toxins, bacteria, and other cytokines such as IL-1β.[19]

High levels of TNFα sounds like something we don't want. Truth is, TNFα is a critical part of our immune system. Low levels can result in *cachexia*, or wasting syndrome, which manifests as drastic weight loss, muscle atrophy, fatigue, weakness, and significant loss of appetite.

Instead of finding out why these cytokines are elevated in the first place, or looking at the intricate interactions of hundreds of other hormones that could be at play, doctors simply treat the problem with TNFα blockers.

In fact—and this makes me particularly angry—they started using TNFα blockers to see what they would do in HS patients *before having evidence that TNFα was actually even present in HS skin*.[20] Nice. Doesn't that give you a warm, fuzzy feeling inside?

One Doctor's Take
Symptoms are the body's warning signals of trouble from within. Taking a medication designed to simply suppress the symptoms of a disease without addressing the root cause, could be likened to turning off the fire alarm while your house burns. Adding fuel to the flames are the unavoidable side effects and toxicity of most pharmaceutical medications.

—Dr. Ronald Drucker, *The Code of Life*

When TNFα blockers actually worked in some people, researchers set about to find out why. That's when they discovered that TNFα actually *is* elevated in HS skin.[21] You heard me right: they gave us these powerful drugs without knowing how, why, or if they would work in the first place.

So it turns out the medication *did* work in a select few individuals. What's the problem? Why aren't we *all* on TNFα blockers? Back in 2011, the FDA notified healthcare professionals that the boxed warning for the entire class of TNFα blockers had been updated to include the risk of infection from legionella and listeria, two potentially deadly bacterial pathogens. The FDA also advised that patients treated with TNFα blockers are at "increased risk for developing serious infections involving multiple organ systems that may lead to hospitalization or death due to bacterial, mycobacterial, fungal, viral, parasitic, and other opportunistic pathogens."[22] Fan-freakin-tastic.

But wait—that's not all.

In order to avoid reactivation of latent tuberculosis, doctors are supposed to administer a purified protein derivative test before prescribing TNFα blockers. If you take them, there is also the risk of anaphylaxis, the formation of human antichimeric antibodies, delayed hypersensitivity reactions, the risk of lymphoproliferative disease, and drug-induced lupus.[23] I'm not going to explain all those things, but suffice it to say, you don't want any of them to happen to you or anyone you love.

These drugs mess with your immune system big time. *If* they work, it can take over a year to see any effect. Plus, they don't deal with *all* the pro-inflammatory cytokines present in HS lesional skin—*only* with TNFα. They also don't get to the root of the problem—*why* these inflammatory cytokines are elevated in the first place. They simply block your body from producing an important component of the immune response.

TNFα blockers include Remicade (infliximab), Enbrel (etanercept), Humira (adalimumab), Cimzia (certolizumab pegol), and Simponi (golimumab). If your doctor suggests any of these medications for you to take, consider yourself warned.

"YOU NEED TO TAKE ANTIANDROGENS OR BIRTH CONTROL PILLS."
Early studies on HS found that patients with HS almost always have excess androgen (testosterone) levels. If HS is caused by excess testosterone, then blocking that testosterone should solve the problem, right? Wrong. Blocking androgens only covers up the symptoms. It doesn't solve the problem—and it can actually create new ones. It doesn't work forever, either. As your body struggles to find balance, other hormones can go out of whack, either resulting in a relapse or a whole new set of symptoms for you to enjoy.

Antiandrogen medications, like *cyproterone acetate*, compete with testosterone for androgen receptors on cells and also reduce the amount of testosterone your body makes by creating a negative feedback effect on the hypothalamic-pituitary-gonadal (HPG) axis.[24] This axis is responsible for development, reproduction, and aging. Fluctuations in hormones controlled by the HPG axis can cause changes in hormones produced by other glands. This results in both widespread and local effects on the body. In the case of antiandrogen medications, these effects can include

LEISH'S STORY

Ten years ago, they started small, right on the crease of my boob. Oh boy, they were small but SO painful. They were only coming up I'd say every three months, but getting bigger each time. About a year after this started, my grandfather passed away and I had the biggest one ever. I had to go to hospital because the pain was unbearable. I had to actually get put under and have minor surgery. The surgeon told me he got a half a pint of puss out, which led me to ask, "What are they, why am I getting these?" His response was, "We live in a tropical area and you sweat under there."

After two weeks of the build up of this massive abscess, I had to take another week off work just to recover. I remember it wasn't long before I felt another come up. They were coming more frequently, and going from one boob to the next. So I went to a lady doctor, who I felt comfortable with, she would give me a local antiseptic, and lance it. But I could feel it OH MY GOD, I would scream. Then she would try to put a "wick" in it, to keep it open to let all the pus out. I sit here and shake my head now, remembering the pain I suffered.

Leish, 33
North Queensland, Australia

decreased muscle mass, loss of libido and attention, increased abdominal fat, impotence, and increased risk of fractures.

Sometimes birth control pills are prescribed as a way to introduce extra estrogen, which can improve HS symptoms by decreasing the amount of free testosterone in the blood.[25] However, even birth control pills themselves are not without dangerous side effects.

Birth control pills have a very similar effect on our gut flora as antibiotics. They contain synthetic hormones, which can change the way that insulin responds to glucose and increase the risk of cardiovascular disease, blood clots, and stroke.[26] Birth control pills may even contain alkaloids or other gut-irritating ingredients that are not listed on the package.

Some women take birth control for unrelated matters, like irregular periods, endometriosis, polycystic ovary syndrome (PCOS), premenstrual syndrome (PMS), or premenstrual dysphoric disorder (PMDD), and find some relief from their HS. I was on the pill for more than fourteen years, and I can tell you that it had no effect whatsoever on *my* HS, though it did regulate my periods, clear my acne, and seem to improve my PMS symptoms. While on the pill, my HS went into severe stage II. When I eventually stopped taking the pill, I discovered it had been masking some pretty serious conditions that I had been previously unaware of—like PCOS and endometriosis. There are many reasons to be on the pill and only you can decide if it is worth the risk. But don't fool yourself into thinking that extra estrogen will cure you.

Female HS patients are often prescribed a medication called *spirono-lactone* (brand names Aldactone and Spirotone) if they complain of flare-ups right before their period. Spironolactone is used to treat many different problems, from high blood pressure to fluid retention. It is not recognized by the FDA as an acne treatment and has not been shown to reduce acne in clinical trials. However, there is some evidence that spironolactone reduces excessive hair growth.[27] The medical term for excessive hair growth is *hirtuism*, and it's caused by increased sensitivity to androgens in the hair follicles. If our pores are clogged from excess progesterone and our hair is growing excessively from too much testosterone, it can result in a pimple or a boil.

Spironolactone's primary use is as an aldosterone antagonist. It prevents your body from absorbing too much salt and keeps your potassium levels from getting too low by blocking the important hormone aldosterone.

There is no clinical evidence that spironolactone is effective for HS, but it continues to be prescribed. Aldosterone is an important hormone and if you take a medication to block its production, there are consequences. The side effects of low aldosterone just happen to be exactly the same as the side effects of spironolactone: thirst, dry mouth, stomach cramps, excess sweating, headache, dizziness, increased blood potassium levels, and low blood pressure. Spironolactone can also cause irregular periods and breast tenderness.

If you suspect that excess testosterone is playing a part in your HS flare-ups, check out chapter five, *The Hormone Connection*, where we'll learn natural ways to get your hormones back in balance.

> Fifty percent of all doctors graduate in the bottom half of their class. Hope your surgery went well!
>
> —Simone Elkeles, *Rules of Attraction*

They May Suggest Surgery

Once the antibiotics fail (as they typically do), the next option your doctor will suggest is surgery. In this regard, they are treating the condition much the same way you would treat cancer: you cut it out. Trouble is, when you simply remove an organ, gland, or piece of tissue that is being ravaged by an *autoimmune response*, it doesn't stop that autoimmune response from happening elsewhere. All your *other* organs, glands, and tissues are now open to attack.

HS surgery is invasive. It can take over two years to fully heal from it. During that time, you may be immobilized even more than you were before. There is also no guarantee that the surgery will be a success. The statistics are not in your favor—you have an over 80 percent chance of having immediate flare-ups in the *exact same place* if the surgery isn't done correctly.[28]

There appears to be a right way and a wrong way of performing HS surgery. The **wrong** way is to lance the boil, cut into the boil, or to try and cut the boil out and stitch it up. The surgeon will refer to this as "incision" or "excision and subsequent primary closure."

The **right** way is with "wide excision and subsequent secondary healing or split-skin grafting." Depending on where you live, the doctor may also refer to this as a *debridement*. Essentially, the surgeon cuts open a wide area and scars it by removing all the skin, hair follicles, and glands. "As scars are free from hair and glands," Dr. von der Werth writes, "the disease is deprived of its core structures."[29] That is to say, no glands or hair follicles equals no place for boils to form.

If you are undergoing the subsequent secondary healing procedure, your body will eventually grow scar tissue over the surgical area. If you opt for the split-skin grafting, surgeons will take skin from somewhere else on your body known as a donor area. The new skin will be grafted over the surgical area.

There is the chance that a skin graft will fail—in other words, the new skin can die. You will also have to simultaneously heal in the donor area, which is usually more painful than the surgical site itself.

Scarring is extensive with this type of surgery, but that's kind of the point: scarring has been found to be the *only* type of surgery that is effective for HS. Since HS boils scar quite badly themselves, the scars

> Isn't it a bit unnerving that doctors call what they do "practice?"
>
> —George Carlin

from surgery can equate to "six of one, half a dozen of the other" to many sufferers. If your HS is severe and the doctor suggests debridement, or wide excision and subsequent secondary healing, or split-skin grafting, read about what to expect in *Kiley's Story* featured in this chapter.

If you're still unsure whether HS surgery is for you, google "hidradenitis" and "surgery." There are tons of stories online about people who went under the knife and had reoccurrences of their HS—often in the same place, *while still healing*. There are also stories of people who had successful procedures with no more reoccurrences in the surgical area. I've yet to hear of someone who has had his or her HS go into remission because of surgery.

Sometimes flare-ups are so bad—and so constant—surgery really feels like the only way out. I don't blame anyone in stage III for having it done; I can imagine the pain that ultimately leads to making such a drastic decision. If you are currently considering surgery, understand that it will take care of only the boils you have *right now*. It won't stop new ones from popping up somewhere else later on.

And finally, make sure you have a damned good doctor and give yourself at least a couple months to recover. It is imperative that you make sure your surgeon is up to date on what works—and what doesn't—before you go under the knife.

"WE CAN SCAR THE AREA WITH CRYOTHERAPY OR COLD LASER THERAPY"

Scarring can also be achieved with aggressive cryotherapy or cold laser therapy. In cryotherapy, your skin is exposed to subzero temperatures or liquid nitrogen. This is normally done to remove warts. There is the risk that the skin in the area may turn white or die, although if properly done, it should only blister.

Do not have you doctor attempt to freeze off a particularly painful boil as if it were a wart. If your doctor suggests this, run away. Von der Werth advises that cryotherapy should be limited to only the most chronically inflamed areas of disease and should be avoided for the majority of HS lesions, that is, the self-limiting boils that run their course without treatment.[30] But you must wait until you are clear of lesions and then proceed to scar the area. Theoretically no more boils can form there.

Keep in mind that relief is not immediate. It can take anywhere from eight to thirty treatments before there is any type of relief. You should also have a lengthy consultation with the doctor who is going to perform the operation to make sure she understands what HS is. The procedures are not typically covered by insurance.

What about laser hair removal?

If stage I and II HS affects the hair follicle, it makes sense that removing the hair would make it stop, right?

In theory, yes, it does make sense. However, laser hair removal doesn't remove the hair follicle; it only removes the *hair* in that follicle. Eventually, that hair will grow back.

I searched online for testimonies from people who had tried this to see if it worked. I found a blog dedicated to HS and laser hair removal, complete with lots of pictures and details about the procedure. The young woman who wrote it was very open about all the different medications she had tried, and posted pictures and descriptions every single time she went to the doctors.

The problem is, her last post is from January 2010. She also mentions being on a special type of birth control pill that cuts down the number of periods you have to four times a year. She reports losing weight as well. It's unclear whether the laser hair removal, the weight loss, or the medication is what's working for her. There isn't any contact information on the site, so I can't reach out and see how she's doing. I am not optimistic that laser hair removal alone would work long term. This is her last post:

> My HS is still doing really good. I get about 1–2 nodules every 6 months. I still need to keep getting laser hair removal every 6 months when my hair starts to grow back more. But I have really dark thick hair so it's hard for the lasers to ever completely and permanently get rid of all the hair. It's still completely worth it though; monetarily wise it's only $150 a year. My happiness is worth that and more. —http://aenigma20.blogspot.com

Laser hair removal is very painful and can be expensive. It won't make the HS go away forever nor will it put you into remission. However, it may give you some temporary relief in the area that you have the procedure done.

A few final thoughts on surgery

Dr. von der Werth advises that patients should remember that surgery—even extensive surgery—can never cure HS and warns that the disease may erupt again outside of the operation area at a later stage.[31]

Never feel pressured to go under the knife because your doctor tells you it is your only option. Your doctor is not the one who has to heal from the surgery: YOU are. Only you can make this decision. If you feel pressured or coerced, or are not given answers that satisfy you before you undergo the operation, find another doctor.

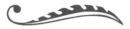

Kiley's Story

I've included many personal stories in this book, but none has touched me as much as Kiley's. She is a stage III HS patient who has had a really rough go of things and blogs about her experience with HS at NotDying.wordpress.com, where, in addition to her personal stories, she shares interviews with medical professionals and the latest medical advancements on HS.

Kiley has had several surgeries for her HS and despite severe flare-ups and set backs, keeps an amazingly positive attitude. Here is the story of the surgeries she underwent in 2012:

By the time I walked into the elective surgery unit for the second time in a little under three months, I felt like an old war hero returning to the battlefield. I walked through the crisscrossed hallways, and nodded and waved to those on staff that I recognized from my previous forays onto the quiet ward.

My previous surgery had been an entirely different ordeal. Three months before, I had officially reached stage III hidradenitis—or, as it is otherwise known, "the bad stage." (Although, none of the stages are particularly good, to be honest.)

I arrived at the hospital for my first surgery reserved and quiet. I was afraid of everything, as I had never really been in a hospital before. The procedure that I was to have, the surgeon informed me, was called a "debridement." A debridement is where they remove diseased and/or damaged skin. They do it for myriad reasons, including bacterial infection, skin diseases, and tumorous conditions. For HS, it is the last, most extreme step to take, when every other avenue has been exhausted.

As I said before, I was terrified of everything—the anesthetic, the surgery itself, and the recovery. I stared around the room with wide, unblinking eyes, unable to even force up a smile for the nurses that took my blood pressure and temperature every fifteen minutes. The surgeon arrived and began to describe in detail exactly what he was going to do. Basically, he was going to carve me open like a Christmas turkey and then scoop out everything. And I mean, everything—hair, skin, fat, it would all be gone—but not just my arm, my right breast, too. I swallowed and nodded. I had accepted in the weeks prior that it needed to be done or I would spend the rest of my life an invalid, unable to move or care for myself.

The rest of the day went by in a nervous blur. I was wheeled into the operating room, and the anesthesiologist gave me a shot of something. They put a mask on me and I was out.

When I came to in a private room, they had a loose dressing on my arm in preparation for something called a wound VAC. A wound VAC is a small vacuum that is attached with a tube and sponges to wounds. It encourages healing via suction.

This meant that I could see what had just been done clearly in the daylight of the hospital room. Nauseous, I could see where the sharpness of the scalpel had sliced away my rotten, diseased flesh, and as my eyes traveled a little further, I felt something catch in my throat. It took a few moments to register what exactly had been done but as it did, I realized that almost the entire side of my breast had been completely removed. It looked so odd—like ... like the edge of a cliff, where the land just ceases to be—my flesh, quite similarly, had just ceased to *be*.

I took a deep breath and composed myself, remembering that the surgeon had said that the year ahead would be a long and tough road, fit only for those that possessed the stamina to go through all of the needed steps. I had agreed to the upcoming challenge rather quickly that day, never knowing I would ever feel an ounce of despair at my now distorted, disfigured body.

A tiny voice of reason spoke quietly from a dark corner of my brain:

Wasn't your body disfigured before?

Well, yes.

And how do you feel now?

I thought for a moment, searching for the stinging coiled pain of hidradenitis suppurativa beneath my skin, which had become so familiar, so expected, over the past three years.

After a minute or two I was still searching for it ...

And my smile suddenly returned. It wasn't there.

The couple of months that followed where rough, but before I knew it, I was off the wound VAC and visiting my surgeon for a progress check.

"So," he said, "we still have the left arm to work on, yes?"

"That's right, yes," I said.

"How does next Tuesday sound? I had a cancellation."

"Uhh," I stammered, my mouth dry. "Sure, OK, yeah. Let's go for it."

"Excellent! Now, that side is not as bad as your other one was, so I will be doing a slightly different procedure."

I found out later that the procedure was a form of "deroofment," or removing the top layer of skin. It has a high rate of success among HS sufferers.

Back on the ward, before the second surgery was to begin, the staff began to admit all the people that were having surgery that day. The staff and I were practically on a first-name basis by then, so I had quite a few nurses and orderlies around my bed, chatting—sort of like a morbid celebrity, I suppose.

The head nurse pulled the privacy curtain closed around my bed and began to change the dressings of my previous surgical wound. They called in a student nurse to watch, and that's when she began my tale of woe. "Ach!" she said, in an accent that I was convinced was Scottish but everyone tells me is "culchie." "Ya shoolda seen the poor thing right when she come outta surgery! The incision was 30 centimeters wide, if it was a mile! Aye, you could put your fist all tha way through!" She demonstrated by putting her fist through her other hand.

"It's true," said an orderly, a young man with a head full of white hair. "And the smell! Oh, God, the smell! We could smell you coming down the hall! It was dreadful!"

I laughed. I couldn't help it. I knew he wasn't trying to be offensive and, actually, he was quite accurate. Besides, I liked him, as he had always been good for a nice bit of gossip on my previous visits.

After all the ooing and ahhing was done, I was left to my own devices for a while, since my surgery wasn't scheduled until late that afternoon. I tried to relax and take a few deep breaths to calm my nerves. Despite knowing that the arm that was due to be operated on was far less damaged than the other one had been, I was still worried about what was coming up. Fear of the unknown, I suppose.

I watched as a Presbyterian minister and a nun came to the ward and visited their respective patients, each offering similar prayers and words of comfort. I watched family members arrive and leave. I watched mounds of paperwork being filled out. I watched as each bed was wheeled out one by one, and the room grew quieter, until it was my turn.

The head nurse walked alongside my bed, helping one of the orderlies push it to the operating room. They parked me just inside the crash doors and she said, "Well, don't take this the wrong way, but I hope this is the last time we ever meet, my dear!" She shook my hand and gave me a smile before walking out.

I lay there, staring up at the familiar ceiling, the giant light shining right in my eyes and heard another voice say, "Hey, haven't you been here before?"

"Yes," I said nervously, my stomach beginning to churn so hard that it would make the Amish envious.

The anesthesiologist, this one different from the one I'd had previously, roughly shoved an oxygen mask at me. "Here, take this. Breathe. I don't want you passing out before we knock you out." She was gruff, her language clipped and blunt.

They transferred me from the bed to the narrow operating table. Five million different people ran around doing five million different things at once—and yet, they were oddly synchronized. The anesthesiologist slapped at my hand, as another lady put a blood pressure cuff on me. The anesthesiologist growled, "You have terrible veins ... and the fact that I have only one hand to work with really narrows down my choices!"

Yeah, well, that's your problem, lady, not mine.

She stuck a needle in my forearm and began to dig around, I felt the room start to spin as she did, and I took deep, measured breaths from the mask on my face.

When I came to in the recovery room, I noticed immediately that my hospital ID bracelet had been cut and taped to my hand and a new IV spot had been inserted onto the side of it. I also very quickly noted that I was in massive pain and, as my eyes focused, I moaned to the nurse, "I hurt. A lot. Lots of pain, I'm not kidding."

Now, I'll be honest here, I've been kicked in the head multiple times while kick-boxing and kneed in the ribs more than a normal person probably ever should be—and I had also already been through a massive debridement of skin on my right side that was removed all the way down to the muscle—and none of it even came close to mirroring the pain that I was in when I awoke.

Upon noticing my eyes were open, a student surgeon ambled over with a smile and told me, "Well, good news. We didn't have to remove that much skin after all!"

"Is it as deep as the muscle?" I tried to ask between gasps.

"Oh, no! This is completely superficial!" she exclaimed.

"Is that why it hurts so much?"

She nodded sympathetically. "Probably, yeah. Sorry about that." She gave me a wink and a pat on the shoulder and ambled back away.

I hated her at that moment. Very much. With everything inside of me.

Over the next twenty-five minutes they pumped me full of as much morphine as they were allowed, but it did very little in the way of easing any of my pain—so they gave me a few of my favorite little white, round friends: codeine. Only then, about forty-five minutes after waking up, did my pain begin to recede.

That night was rough.

But before long it had ended and when morning came again, I noticed that I was in very little pain. In fact, for the first time in two years, my left arm had no pain in a resting position. I was very happy with this development and couldn't wait for my surgeon to visit.

Which he did, about an hour later. He explained to me that he hadn't taken much away and that the tunneling was very light on that side, so he didn't have to go very deep either. He also said that since I had handled the dressing change without much discomfort, I could go home later.

It's now been six months since the last surgery, and while I'm still healing from the first, the second has failed. I will be returning for further surgery on my left arm and also again, later in the year, for new surgeries on my groin, as they are both affected by stage II HS.

As for my right arm, I still have a long way to go, as years of holding my arms at my sides, bent at the elbows like a horribly disease-afflicted Barbie doll, have reprogrammed my mind. I still baby my right arm, although there isn't any reason to, and I still hesitate to reach for things, although there is no pain to speak of when I do.

I suppose, like everything, it's a learning process but I am happy to be going through it.

After I received this story from Kiley, I wrote to her and asked her some more questions. It had been just a little more than a year since her surgery. As with any other treatment for HS, sufferers are very interested to know how things work out in the long run.

How long have you had HS? I had stage I from the age of twelve and then developed stage II about two years ago and crashed headlong into stage III a little over a year ago—so nearly twenty years! Yeesh! I've never done the math before!

Can you tell us a little more about the surgery? The surgeon did a deroofing procedure, which has been proven fantastic for most sufferers but, unfortunately, it just opened up all those sinus tracts and they multiplied like crazy!

What's next for you? Are you going to have any more surgeries? Right now the plan is to do a debridement with a skin graft and wound VAC therapy afterwards. The surgeon says he may have to adapt his ideas once he's in there.

How long did it take you to heal from your first surgery? Technically, I'm not healed. I still have an open little area on my under arm and one on my breast. It's been exactly one year and one week since the first surgery.

Did the surgery help? In individual areas, I'd say some of it got worse but collectively, overall, I seemed to improve for a few months—less flares, better movement, etc.—but then as the individual sites have gotten worse, everything has started to tumble back downhill.

Overall, how are things? There is still a wound [under my right arm], although it is significantly smaller than before. The surgery [under my left arm] failed, I think it's still technically stage II. I also have wounds on my ears now. It's a kind of rarely affected area.

Kiley is a source of inspiration for many in the HS community. She is a published author who grew up in Texas, but who now lives in Belfast, N. Ireland. You can read more about her battle with HS at NotDying. wordpress.com.

CHAPTER THREE
Autoimmunity 101

It is no measure of health to be well adjusted to a profoundly sick society.
—Jiddu Krishnamurti

e've talked a lot about what HS isn't. Now let's get down to business and discuss what it actually *is*.

Hidradenitis suppurativa is an autoimmune disease. Autoimmune diseases are nasty, complicated things. A cure—not to mention a standardized treatment—for autoimmunity has long eluded the minds of some of the most brilliant research scientists and doctors. Billions of dollars have been spent on research. Debate about the cause of these horrible diseases continues to plague the scientific community. I believe the researchers are looking in the wrong place. They are trying to find a magic pill. The answer lies elsewhere.

According to progressive doctors, recent scientific studies, and experts in the Primal/paleo community, *leaky gut syndrome* is the likely culprit behind autoimmune conditions.[1] People from all over the world have reported that once they healed their guts, they regained their health and vitality. These are people who once suffered from debilitating autoimmune diseases like multiple sclerosis and rheumatoid arthritis. Not only have they put their diseases into remission, they've actually *reversed* damage to their bodies that they were told was permanent.

They are healed. And they did it on their own, without medication or surgery. However, because these are personal experiences and not documented, official, scientific studies, the media and your doctor have not picked up on them. Yet.

We are still learning much about the human body, and there are still many things that we don't know. For instance, we don't know why some people with autoimmunity present different symptoms. No one can tell you why you have HS affecting your armpits and your brother has it in his groin.

That said, this chapter is going to answer a lot of questions you have about the nature of HS: why there are periods of remission, why it migrates, why an effective treatment has escaped the medical community for so long, and why it keeps coming back no matter what you do.

By the time you finish reading this chapter, it will all make sense. It will be *so obvious* that you're dealing with autoimmunity, you may even feel angry with yourself for not figuring it out earlier. Don't be. There is no power in *what could have been*. There is only power in *what is*.

So before you barge into your doctor's office and demand to know why *they* didn't know this stuff, what with all their book learnin' and fancy degrees, please consider that your doctor has likely been trained to dispense medication rather than nutrition advice. It isn't your doctor's fault. It's the system. Your doctor likely doesn't know …

- that HS is an autoimmune response
- how to mitigate an autoimmune response without medication
- what causes autoimmunity
- how diet affects the body

Soon, you will know all of this and more. Keep reading.

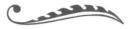

How HS Manifests

In 2011, I was lucky enough to meet Dr. Loren Cordain. He is a renowned researcher specializing in evolutionary medicine, one of the world's leading experts on the Paleolithic diet, and the author of many books on the subject. I asked him point blank about hidradenitis suppurativa and what he thought about it. I figured if anyone in this world knew what was going on, it would be him. I was right. Cordain was the first (and only) doctor to ever utter the words "hidradenitis" and "autoimmunity" in the same sentence to me. He'd seen enough evidence—both clinical and anecdotal—to convince him that HS is autoimmune in nature. Here's an excerpt from his popular blog, ThePaleoDiet.com:

> Abundant scientific evidence exists in hidradenitis suppurativa (HS) patients showing that pro-inflammatory cytokines (local hormones) are elevated in the blood [and] are almost certainly involved in the skin lesions presenting in HS patients. Two major categories of circulating white blood cells (macrophages and dendritic cells) likely have become activated (sensitized) in the gut to specific gut proteins (either bacteria or food or both) and these gut-borne cells then initiate an immune response that affects cell lining, either the hair follicle or apocrine sweat glands in other parts of the body (particularly the groin and armpit areas). Hence, it seems likely that HS, although it presents clinically as a single disease, is actually at least two diseases (one in the hair follicle and one in the apocrine sweat glands)—both likely to be autoimmune in nature.[2]

Let's translate. First, you'll remember from the last chapter that cytokines are chemical messengers in our blood that are made by immune cells. A high level of cytokines in your blood means your body thinks it's under attack and is launching an immune response. And, as you may recall, HS boils and lesions have been shown to have high levels of inflammatory cytokines.[3] This is our first connection between HS and autoimmunity.

In addition to this, Cordain says the immune cells in our gut have become sensitive to proteins from certain foods or bacteria. These immune cells launch an attack (autoimmune response) whenever these proteins (our "triggers") are present. Coupled with the inflammation from the cytokines, this creates a pretty nasty outcome for us. The immune response affects the cells lining our hair follicles (or our sweat glands when inflammation is very great).

But here's the kicker: Cordain proposes that HS is not just *one* disease, split up into three stages, but is actually *two* separate diseases—one in the hair follicles and one in the apocrine (sweat) glands. This would certainly explain why some people present immediately in stage III and why others never get there.

According to Cordain, women are more likely to have the form of HS that involves the cells lining the hair follicle. That's why you may see hairs trapped within the boils or why you may have thought you had a really bad ingrown hair problem. If, however, you are dealing with the form that affects your sweat glands, chances are you have already been diagnosed with severe stage III HS.

Back in 2002 Cordain's research group, along with a separate group led by renowned celiac researcher Alessio Fasano at the University of Maryland, discovered evidence that suggests that leaky gut is a key triggering event in most autoimmune diseases.[4] And Cordain's suggestion for all autoimmune patients? Restrict foods known to increase intestinal permeability. That's the scientific term for leaky gut.

In the next chapter, we'll look more closely at leaky gut syndrome, what causes it, and how to heal from it. But for now, let's get a basic understanding of what exactly autoimmunity is.

The Basics

Autoimmune diseases develop when your immune system gets confused and can't tell the difference between it's own tissues and invading organisms. Your immune system essentially misfires and attacks your own tissue as if it were the bad guys. Since your immune system is confused, it starts to destroy perfectly good tissue, resulting in pain and suffering in the form of a disease, for which there is seemingly no cause or cure.

An autoimmune attack creates multiple forms of inflammation, tissue damage, pain, and cascading imbalances, which may involve any and all organs and bodily systems.[5] It can manifest as practically anything—from dandruff to lupus.

In his popular book *The Paleo Diet*, Cordain discusses something called molecular mimicry. He writes:

Surprisingly, we have found that many common gut bacteria fragments are made up of the same molecular building blocks as those found in certain immune system proteins and in the tissue under attack by the immune system.

This confuses the immune system to no end. Through this process of molecular mimicry, milk, grain, legume, and nightshade proteins can trick the immune system into attacking the body's own tissues.[6]

Autoimmune diseases used to be pretty rare. Nowadays they seem to be commonplace. We're discovering that many health conditions we didn't know were autoimmune actually are. Diabetes, asthma, endometriosis, and restless leg syndrome used to be something you just "got," while the label "autoimmune" was reserved for the likes of lupus and multiple sclerosis (MS).

If you were to survey all the known autoimmune conditions, it's hard to find someone these days who isn't somehow affected. People are becoming sicker than ever before, and the trend appears to be nowhere in decline. In fact, incidences of diabetes, asthma, endometriosis, and other autoimmune diseases are higher today than ever before.

The medical industry refers to many of these conditions as "diseases of aging" and tells us that they are just a normal part of life. We're told these conditions

THE IMMUNE SYSTEM

Your immune system is an intricate and effective network. Millions of cells—organized like a powerful army—pass information back and forth to each other. When a foreign invader is detected, entire regiments of your immune system army mobilize and prepare to attack.

As the cells mobilize, they produce powerful chemicals that allow other cells to grow, enlist their fellow soldiers, and direct new recruits to combat areas—then off to war they go.

Usually this is a good thing, like when we catch a virus or a cold. But when it's overloaded with threats and enemies, your immune system's delicate network starts misfiring; there's just no way to keep up a war on all fronts, at all times.

In a posttraumatic stress disorder-fueled haze, your immune system starts seeing everything as the enemy—especially certain foods you eat, because their proteins are detected in places they shouldn't be, namely your bloodstream. So, your immune system, not sure who the real enemy is anymore, mounts a counterattack and starts creating cells and antibodies directed against your tissues. This friendly fire can affect any part of your body, and it can destroy many parts of your body at the same time. This is autoimmunity.

are incurable or that the cause is unknown. The only thing we can do is treat the symptoms.

Most of the time, the person suffering is unaware that all their symptoms are autoimmune in nature. Unnecessary—yet profit-able—surgeries are often preformed. The diseased organ or tissue is removed, leaving the autoimmunity free to attack other organs and tissues. If the patient gets worse, the doctor often prescribes immune suppressing drugs. No mention is ever made of restoring proper immune system function.[7] If you're now left wondering why the medical community seems to have its head up its ass, ponder for a moment these words taken from Dr. Ronald Drucker's book, *The Code of Life*:

> Through appointments, tests, drugs, and surgical procedures, autoimmunity generates and represents an estimated 85 percent of the revenue collected by the medical and pharmaceutical complex in total. Without autoimmunity, this massive bureaucratic industry would be restricted to generating revenue from little more than pregnancies and trauma accidents.

The Name of the Game

If you have autoimmunity, the disease you end up with depends on what your immune system attacks. Writes Cordain in *The Paleo Diet*:

> When the immune system invades and destroys nerve tissue, multiple sclerosis and other neurological diseases develop. When the pancreas is the target, type-1 diabetes occurs. When joint tissues are attacked and destroyed, the result is rheumatoid arthritis.[8]

The skin is the largest organ in the human body,[9] although, since it's located outside the body, we tend not to think of it as an "organ." Regardless of how we choose to think about it, our skin is made up of a complex system of glands, cell layers, and nerves, and it is in constant contact with the rest of our body. We already know that autoimmune disease targets the skin in many forms, including psoriasis and dermatitis herpetiformis,[10] so it makes sense that it could target the skin in the form of hidradenitis suppurativa.

Take a look at this chart. Can you tell what all the diseases and conditions listed below have in common?

WHEN AUTOIMMUNITY ATTACKS...	THE RESULT IS CALLED...
Blood and Blood Vessels	anemia, lupus, Wegener's granulomatosis.
Tear Ducts or Saliva Glands	Sjogren's syndrome
Thyroid Gland	Hashimoto's thyroiditis, Grave's disease
Kidneys	glomerulonephritis, lupus, type-1 diabetes, mellitus
Joints	arthritis (all kinds)
Muscles	fibromyalgia, myasthenia gravis
Nerves & Brain	multiple sclerosis, Guillain-Barré syndrome
Pancreas	diabetes
Heart	myocarditis, rheumatic fever, scleroderma
Skin	eczema, psoriasis, rosacea, dermatitis herpetiformis, hidradenitis suppurativa, alopecia, vitiligo
Digestive Tract (including Mouth)	autoimmune hepatitis, scleroderma, gastritis, irritable bowel syndrome, acid reflux, GERD, hiatal hernia, Barrett's esophagus
Small Intestinal Tract	Crohn's disease, celiac disease, chronic fatigue syndrome
Colon	ulcerative colitis, diverticulosis, diverticulitis
Multiple Areas of the Body Simultaneously	lupus (joints, skin, kidneys, blood cells, heart and lungs)

Table 1. Sources: Dr. Ronald P. Drucker, Dr. Loren Cordain, www.diseases.EMedTV.com

This is not an exhaustive list of autoimmune conditions, but it paints a pretty good picture. The root problem of all these (and other) conditions is autoimmunity. *The disease itself is autoimmunity*. How that disease manifests in you is what the doctors will diagnose you with. Make sense?

The diagnosis—let's say, arthritis or IBS—is simply a term that identifies the result of an autoimmune attack on a specific area of the body. Dr. Ronald Drucker writes in *The Code Of Life* that…

> The medical doctor has no motive to educate or discuss this with the patient, for they are trained to treat symptoms only and have no reason to discuss the root cause. They are taught by the system that the root cause—autoimmunity—is incurable…. And in most cases, the doctors are unaware that various conditions and symptoms alike are autoimmune or autoimmune related.[11]

If It Walks Like a Duck

If you look at a list of known autoimmune diseases,[12] you will see a few things they all have in common. For one, they are listed as chronic, meaning that these diseases last a long, long time, sometimes forever. Second, there are no known cures. And third, they may be described as having no known cause other than being autoimmune. A lot of the time, no standardized treatment exists for these diseases because there is no treatment that works particularly well.

Sounds a lot like HS, doesn't it?

There are over a hundred known autoimmune conditions and hundreds of autoimmune symptoms, but something most autoimmune issues have in common is inflammation. In HS, the inflammation is apparent in the boils. Hard to miss, really. In other autoimmune issues, the inflammation is hidden in places like your joints (arthritis), your nerves (multiple sclerosis) or your colon (ulcerative colitis).

To make the cascading effect of autoimmunity a little easier to understand, Robb Wolf, author of *The Paleo Solution*, says to "think about the full immune system like a civil defense force in that if one section of the defense force is on alert or active, all elements are on higher alert."[13] That's why you may flare up when you are stressed, when you get your period, when you're sick, or when you eat sugar.

Why Me? Three Words: Genes, Gut, Environment

Autoimmunity develops in response to three things: the genes you inherited, a leaky gut, and at least one environmental factor. An environmental factor can be a viral or bacterial infection, but the most common is exposure to a certain food.[14,15] These three things—genes, gut, and environment—are known as the holy trinity of autoimmune disease. Until recently, no one knew exactly how autoimmune diseases developed in genetically susceptible people, but Cordain's research points to Neolithic foods such as grains, legumes, dairy products, and nightshades such as potatoes [16] as some of those pesky environmental factors.

Wolf writes that "not only do we have science to support this, we have observed clinical resolution of these conditions upon the removal of grains, legumes, and dairy."[17]

THE HOLY TRINITY

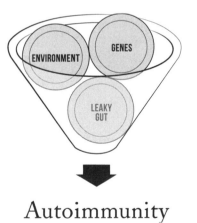

Autoimmunity

In order for your card to come up, the deck has to be stacked a certain way. In other words, you need a combination of genes, certain environmental and dietary factors, and a leaky gut to all come together to create the losing hand. This explains why some people are able to eat or do anything they want without getting sick—maybe they don't have all three factors. It also explains why some families tend to experience disease more than others: why your Aunt Mary has rheumatoid arthritis, your mom has celiac disease, your brother has diabetes, and you have HS.

These are all autoimmune issues, which have manifested themselves in different ways. If this sounds like you and your family, you likely all inherited the genetic component. You also probably all eat the same types of food and have similar attitudes when it comes to taking medications. Chances are, your family history is riddled with disease, chronic illnesses, and unexplained conditions.

We've been told since birth that we are all special and unique, like snowflakes. And there is some truth to that, at least when it comes to your immune systems. A combination of factors such as diet, lifestyle, inflammation, sleep, gut flora, and genetics combine to make your immune system respond differently than your Aunt Mary's.

The good news is we can turn off the autoimmune gene by healing our leaky guts. It's as simple as removing the offending environmental factors, i.e., the offending foods. The trick is finding out which ones. That's where an elimination diet, featured in chapter eight, comes in.

Elimination diets involve removing whole food groups—grains for example—from your diet for a period of time, say two to eight weeks, and then reintroducing them back, one at a time. If removal of a particular food makes you feel better and its reintroduction elicits a negative response, you know you have found one of your triggers. The idea that elimination diets can reduce symptoms of certain diseases is supported by clinical and anecdotal evidence.[18] We know for a fact that there exists a direct link between certain foods and specific diseases. A variety of studies have proved, for example, that gluten causes celiac disease, potatoes aggravate irritable bowel disease, and soy blocks nutrient absorption.

Is There a Cure?

I'm sorry to tell you this, but no, there isn't a definitive *cure* for autoimmunity. A leaky gut, even after it has been healed, causes sensitivity to certain proteins. Even if you take a nice long break from whatever trigger food is causing your disease, if you start eating it again in the future, or don't take care of yourself, the symptoms may come back. In most cases, however, once a person starts healing from leaky gut and is aware of the environmental factors that cause autoimmunity, the symptoms progressively go away.

You can put HS into remission by changing some key factors about your lifestyle. You will have to be fairly diligent about adopting these changes—especially those related to diet. If you stray from the path, your body will let you know loudly and clearly—with inflammation, an HS flare-up, or some other autoimmune response.

One bonus is that if you can keep your key triggers out of your diet for good, you may eventually be able to once again enjoy certain foods—like eggs, coffee, and wine—without flaring up or getting sick. Each and every one of us responds differently to individual foods. You will have to be scientific in your approach and find what works for you.

Remission Defined

Essentially, remission is a lessening of the symptoms of a disease, a temporary reduction, or a complete disappearance. Think of cancer patients just finishing their chemotherapy. If the chemo has killed all of the known cancer and there is no further spread of the disease, the patient is said to be in remission. There is still a chance that the cancer may come back. And what do we call it if it does come back? Relapse. So was the patient ever really in remission? Or was the disease just at such undetectable levels, growing ever so slowly, until it once again presented symptoms? It's great to be optimistic, but sometimes we get carried away before there is enough time to evaluate these things fully.

At the time of publication, there was no standardized definition of the word *remission*. Doctors all over the world mean different things when

AUTOIMMUNE CYCLES

It's bothersome to me when I see people with HS have a two-month remission of their HS and shout out all over the message boards something like this: "Emu oil, turmeric, twelve chili peppers a day, and sweat from a toad collected during the full moon has totally cured my HS!!"

The reason these people think that they have cured themselves of HS is that they don't understand the nature of the disease, in particular the nature of an autoimmune condition. Nor have they truly paid attention to the "cycles" their HS has gone through in the past. It is common for people with autoimmunity to experience periods of remission, sometimes for months at a time, followed by a worsening or lessening of their symptoms, especially if they are exposed to viral or bacterial diseases.[19]

So just because you don't break out for a month doesn't mean you're cured. When you haven't flared up in six months or a year, then we can talk.

they use the word. It has gotten so confusing that doctors at the Childhood Arthritis and Rheumatology Research Alliance (CARRA) held a study[20] to come up with a definite definition for the word—but only where it pertains to pediatric arthritis. I could not find any definitions of the word remission concerning HS. No surprise there.

Since arthritis is an autoimmune response,[21] I believe we can use the criteria from the CARRA Study to define remission as it pertains to other autoimmune conditions, in particular, hidradenitis suppurativa.

The doctors in the CARRA study determined that remission comes in three phases: (1) inactive disease, (2) clinical remission on medication, and (3) clinical remission off medication.

Inactive disease basically means that the disease isn't active. You aren't experiencing any symptoms, and if a doctor were to examine you, he wouldn't find anything.[22]

Only after you have met the criteria for inactive disease for a minimum of six continuous months, can you be considered in a state of clinical remission. If you are using any type of medication to keep yourself in remission, you are considered in a state of clinical remission on medication. The goal is clinical remission off medication. To obtain that lofty ideal, you must meet the criteria for inactive disease for a minimum of twelve continuous months while off all medications.[23]

I am currently in clinical remission off medication. It feels great. It feels like … I'm normal. Any doctor examining me today would not see any signs of HS. I have no flare-ups, pain, or inflammation of any kind. The only telltale sign of HS are a few old scars. I'm not kidding myself, though—I know if I fall off the wagon, my HS will come back with a vengeance. This is why it's called remission, not a cure.

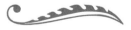

Caveat Emptor

Medical research has found that even after an autoimmune attack sub-sides, varying levels of tissue damage may remain. This depends on the condition and the length of time your body had been under attack. That said, the body has unlimited healing potential, and damaged tissues can be healed and strengthened over time once the attack has subsided. For this to happen, the autoimmune response must be stopped from attack-ing any and all areas of the body.[24] You will have to be patient while your body heals; don't expect complete remission in two weeks. Significant improvement can usually be seen within two to four months. It may take longer for you, but if you haven't seen any improvement at all by the end of 120 days, you will need to reevaluate your approach.

You may also find that once you've removed your triggers for a while, you seem to react more violently to them than you had prior. "Memory cells become attuned or agitated to these peptides so it doesn't take much," explains Cordain. Once you've become sensitized to a certain protein, your immune system stays hypervigilant and even a small dose can cause a major flare-up.[25] This may decrease over time if your body stops producing antibodies to proteins it doesn't come in contact with anymore. However, it's impossible to say for sure that this will happen. It's also fairly ridiculous to think you can completely avoid something as pervasive as gluten for the rest of your life. At some point, you're bound to get inadvertently "dosed" at a restaurant or by a well-meaning family member. And once you've consumed your trigger—knowingly or not—your body will start producing antibodies again.

So there you have it: autoimmunity in a nutshell. Now that you know what it is and recognize HS as being an autoimmune condition, you're well on your way to better health. For more detailed information on autoimmunity, please check out the resource section of this book.

THE SYSTEMS OF THE BODY

We're about to get into some super geeky stuff that you might be tempted to gloss over, but please don't. It's important to know how the systems of your body are connected. In Western medicine, we tend to think of the body's systems as separate unto themselves, compartmentalized into itty-bitty sections instead of looking at the whole picture. It's kind of like going to a department store to look for new bedroom furniture and ending up in Menswear.

The body is made up of ten main systems and several subsystems, which are:

Dermal: skin, hair, nails
Muscular: muscles, tendons
Nervous: brain, spinal cord, nerves
Sensory: eyes, ears, nose, tongue, skin
Endocrine: hormones, glands
Reproductive: penis, testes, ovaries, uterus
Digestive: mouth, pharynx, esophagus, stomach, liver, gall bladder,
    pancreas, small intestine, large intestine, rectum, anus
Circulatory: heart, blood, blood vessels
Lymphatic: tonsils, thymus gland, liver, spleen, lymph nodes
Urinary: kidneys, bladder, urethra
Immune: lymphocytes, antibodies
Skeletal: bones, joints, ligaments, tendons
Respiratory: nose, mouth, pharynx, larynx, trachea, bronchial tubes, lungs
Excretory: skin, lungs, liver, kidneys, large intestine

If you have skin issues, you may see a dermatologist. If you have problems with your nerves, you will see a neurologist. If you have issues with your hormones, they'll send you to an endocrinologist. Bladder problems get you a referral to an urologist. Get the picture? Each one of these doctors specializes in one specific system of the body and each is trained to treat the symptoms of that specific system—nothing more.

In my opinion, seeing a gastroenterologist (a specialist in the digestive system) is a fantastic place to start whenever you have anything wrong with you, because the gut is where most problems start.

CHAPTER FOUR
Follow Your Gut

> *"All disease begins in the gut."*
> —**Hippocrates**

Only in recent years have we begun to associate autoimmunity with leaky gut syndrome. But what exactly is leaky gut? It's every bit as ominous as it sounds: your gut is leaking.

Into your bloodstream.

It's not supposed to do that.

In fact, the body is equipped with a variety of systems designed to prevent just that very thing from happening. But those systems can fail, and when they do, we develop diseases, conditions, and syndromes.

In a healthy gut, toxins, proteins, and bacteria are confined to the intestines until they are eventually released as waste. But if your gut is leaky, some of that waste escapes into your bloodstream.

And that's when the first symptoms appear. Sometimes they present as digestive issues such as constipation or diarrhea, gas, bloating, abdominal pain, heartburn, or irritable bowel syndrome (IBS). Sometimes they aren't so obvious and present as migraines or acne. Unfortunately the first signals our bodies send us indicating something is wrong often go ignored. Our culture is conditioned to think these symptoms are just a normal part of life, and we end up medicating ourselves with over-the-counter drugs. The result is like sticking a Band-Aid on an arterial wound.

Many people with health problems haven't a clue that it's actually their gut giving them issue. In fact, Chris Kresser, a functional medicine practitioner, reports on his health and wellness blog, ChrisKresser.com, that as many as 30 percent of his patients with leaky gut syndrome show no digestive symptoms whatsoever.[1] They are, however, in his office for *something*. This begins to make sense when you consider what happens when the digestive tract starts to break down and function poorly. Essentially, poisons from the gut are carried through the bloodstream to other bodily systems. When these other systems become affected, seemingly unrelated symptoms or diseases suddenly appear from out of nowhere. And to make things more confusing, symptoms differ from person to person, depending on genetic makeup, lifestyle, and the amount of whatever toxin is leaking into the bloodstream.

Approximately 70 percent of those with HS suffer from digestive issues, so the connection between a leaky gut and HS tends to be a little more apparent for us.

Here are a few other symptoms that can show up if your gut is leaky. This is not a complete list, but it shows that leaky gut is often not what we might expect.

- Fatigue
- Joint or muscle aches
- Autoimmune conditions, including HS
- Allergies, hives, rashes, and food allergies
- Depression, mental illness, confusion, and memory loss
- Autism, ADHD, and ADD
- Asthma
- Skin problems, including acne, eczema, psoriasis
- Metabolic problems such as obesity and diabetes
- Inflammation

Speaking of inflammation, it can be an endless cycle: leaky gut causes inflammation in the gut, and inflammation in the gut causes leaky gut, which causes inflammation in the gut, which causes … you get the idea.

You might recall from chapter two, high levels of inflammatory cytokines are found in HS lesions.[2] Why do you think your body produces these cytokines? Because they're reacting to large amounts of toxins that have somehow escaped the gut barrier.[3] This is a natural immune response. As messengers, they travel throughout the body spreading the word of the newly arrived intruders and in turn, create more white blood cells to freak out in your bloodstream. And this creates more inflammation.

Gut Flora and the Gut Barrier

In a healthy person, you'll find more than four hundred different species of bacteria. Some are beneficial and help us break down our food for absorption, and others are harmful and can lead to infection. In total, there are more than 100,000,000,000,000 (100 trillion) microorganisms in a healthy gut, ten times more than all the other cells in the entire human body.[4] That's right, bacteria in our guts outnumber all the other cells in our body by ten to one! When we speak of gut flora, this is what we are talking about. And we're only just beginning to understand the important role it plays in our health.

In addition to regulating metabolism, our gut flora protects the intestinal wall from harmful bacteria and toxins and helps with our digestive processes.

Gut flora also protects us from infection and makes up more than 75 percent of our immune system.[5] (My gastroenterologist says it's more like 85 percent, but either way you get the picture: gut flora's pretty darn important.)

My benchmark for determining whether to run a test [for leaky gut] is whether it will change the outcome of the treatment. Let's say someone comes to me and they have a gut problem. If we were to run a test for leaky gut and it came back and said they didn't have a leaky gut, well, I still have a person with a gut problem. I still need to figure out what's causing that problem and what to do about it. And if someone comes back with a leaky gut, I still need to figure out what's causing it. So there's usually still more work to be done to determine what the underlying cause is.

—Chris Kresser L.Ac,
Revolution Health Radio,
July 2012.

Bad bacteria, toxins, proteins, fragments, and waste also factor into the mix. That's where the good bacteria come in. They keep the bad guys in check. Without a substantial population of good bacteria in the gut, pathogenic bacteria, viruses, yeast, and fungi take over and damage the gut flora's delicate balance. This condition is known as *dysbiosis*, and it basically means that more bad bacteria than good have taken up residence in your gut. Chances are if you have a leaky gut, you have dysbiosis.

In addition to a poor diet, stress, infections, and prescription pills such as birth control pills, painkillers, steroids, and antibiotics are among the many things that can wipe out your beneficial flora. We'll return to our discourse on antibiotics soon, but I want to once again drive home the point how absurd it is that HS patients are, as a first measure, prescribed antibiotics. Studies have shown that antibiotics cause a profound and rapid loss in the diversity of gut flora,[6] and without intervention those beneficial bacteria cannot be recovered.[7]

When antibiotics create such an imbalance, the bad bacteria get nourished every time food enters your gut. They, in turn, excrete toxins that flow into your bloodstream through your ravaged intestinal wall. This leads to illnesses, allergies, and autoimmune reactions. So really what you are getting when you take those antibiotics is a short-term solution that will over time make your HS even worse.

Conversely, if you have healthy gut flora with loads of good bacteria, you may find that you can indulge in your trigger foods from time to time without consequence. You may also find that you fight colds off easier (if you get them at all) and that your health is just generally better.

Another key factor in intestinal health is your gut barrier. We simply cannot discuss it without also mentioning the gastrointestinal (GI) tract, a hollow tube around 30 feet long that passes from your mouth to your anus. It's basically one long mucous membrane covered in various cultures of flora.[8] Those of us with HS have typically experienced some sort of symptom of poor flora *somewhere* along the line: canker sores, chronic strep throat or tonsillitis, acid reflux, abdominal cramps and bloating, or constipation and diarrhea.

Think of the GI track as an interior skin. Its most important function is allowing nutrients in the body while preventing foreign substances from entering. The skin on the outside of our bodies has the exact same job. In fact, our skin really is a mirror of our gut—and vise versa. What happens on the inside is reflected on the outside. So, if you're getting acne, boils, or eczema on the outside, you can bet there is something going on in the inside.

Enzymes and friendly bacteria (if you have any) inside the gut help break down food into their simplest forms. Proteins get broken down into amino acids, carbohydrates into simple sugars, and fats into fatty acids.[9] This, of course, is what our bodies use for fuel. What can't be digested becomes waste.

The gut is also equipped with "gatekeepers." These are highly specialized cells called *enterocytes* that line the gut in a single layer and are responsible for transporting digested nutrients from the intestines into the bloodstream. They are also responsible for keeping everything else in the gut from entering other systems of the body.[10] They are our body's main defense against bacteria, toxins, and unwanted proteins.

When the enterocytes become damaged, they create microscopic holes (or spaces between the cells) through which some of the undesirable contents

ENTEROCYTES: THE GATEKEEPERS

How pathogens made their way into the bloodstream has stumped researchers for years. Under normal circumstances, the gut is fairly impenetrable. Immunologists thought that the enterocytes were "cemented" together with some sort of biological grout. It wasn't until a group of Japanese scientists in the mid-eighties discovered that the spacings between the enterocytes were more similar to a hinge, like one found on a gate door. The enterocytes they found were mostly closed but sometimes open. That's when things started to click. Scientists later found that enterocytes contain tight junctions, that is, proteins that form a tight bond between the enterocytes. It makes sense that if the tight junctions or enterocytes themselves are damaged, anything can pass through—even toxins.[68,69]

of the gut can "leak" out. This allows pathogens that would normally be excreted as waste a passport to explore new and uncharted territory—namely your circulatory system.

The enterocytes aren't the gut's only line of defense. Located immediately outside the gut exist *resident immune cells*, and their job is to protect us against any bad guys that might arbitrarily find their way past the enterocytes. Thanks to both the enterocytes and the resident immune cells, normally only the nutrients from completely digested material gain access into your blood or lymphatic system; however, if your gut is leaky, this isn't the case.

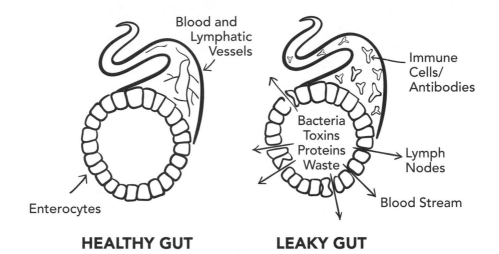

HEALTHY GUT   **LEAKY GUT**

When pathogens leak out of your gut, the resident immune cells recognize them as foreign invaders and mount a response. Exactly what leaks out, and how much, determines the precise nature of the immune response.[11] A continuous, ongoing response ultimately leads to chronic inflammation and autoimmunity. With the systems of your gut barrier failing inside and outside, pathogens that would normally be eliminated as waste now gain access to the circulatory system—a network of blood vessels and lymphatic vessels designed to transport nutrients from the gut to other areas of the body. This explains how those pesky protein fragments, toxins, and bacteria make it all the way from your gut to, say, the cells in your armpits.

The Link Between Neolithic Foods and Leaky Gut

Now that we know what leaky gut is, let's find out why *your* gut is leaking. There's good news and bad news about this one. The good news is, the causes of leaky gut are well documented. Bad news is, they're pretty extensive. Chances are you're going to have to give up some things you take for granted or really enjoy. Trust me when I tell you it will be worth it in the long run.

Quite a lot of research links Neolithic foods with autoimmunity.[12] These are foods that recently entered the human diet. And by "recent," I don't mean March of last year. I mean some ten thousand years ago, when foods like grains, legumes, and dairy were introduced into our diets on a grand scale. Even nightshade vegetables like potatoes, tomatoes, eggplant, and peppers, all products of the New World, were not widely available, if at all.

Our genetic make-up has been shaped by millions of years of evolution. This make-up determines our nutritional and activity needs. Although human genes have remained pretty much unchanged since the agricultural revolution ten thousand years ago, our diet and lifestyle have not. The huge changes our diet and lifestyle have undergone since the Neolithic era, and even more so during the Industrial Revolution, have messed us up big time. In modern Western cultures at least 70 percent of our calories come from foods that were rarely or never consumed by Paleolithic hunter-gatherers.

Doctors James O'Keefe and Loren Cordain state that the mismatch between our modern diet and lifestyle and our Paleolithic genome plays a substantial role in the ongoing epidemics of obesity and disease,[13] and that returning to a Paleolithic-type diet may reduce the risk of many diseases, including cardiovascular disease, metabolic syndrome, diabetes, cancer, acne, and autoimmune conditions.[14]

Now, as for the ole *"Grains have been found at Paleolithic sites!"* and *"There's no way Grok would have passed up milk!"* arguments, think about this: any exposure we had to these foods would have been seasonal and short before the advent of agriculture. If you were susceptible to the proteins in those foods and you started to get sick, chances are you would have run out of the supply of that particular food before you started to develop obesity, autoimmune issues, or cancer. Frankly, autoimmune diseases take time to develop, but given that we have access to Neolithic foods 365 days a year, we have set the stage for them to flourish.

Now let's take a closer look at these everyday modern foods that cause us so much gut ache and grief.

Antinutrients

Grains, legumes, beans, nuts, seeds, and most vegetables contain varying amounts of substances called antinutrients that bind to nutrients and block their absorption into the body. Antinutrients come in the form of lectins, saponins, phytates, and alkaloids, and can have a negative impact on our gut integrity, our immune systems, and our health in general. One of these antinutrients—or a combination of them—may be the cause of your HS.

LECTINS

Lectins are a type of protein found in pretty much all plants, particularly in the seeds. Some plants contain higher amounts than others, so some make us feel sicker than others. Lectins are part of a plant's natural defense system; if its seeds are broken down and digested, they can't grow into new plants. Sometimes a seed will make its way unscathed through the digestive tract of who or whatever ate it and be eliminated intact (in the poop), where it can grow and thrive in nutrient-dense fertilizer. But more often than not, if the seed is eaten, it is destroyed during digestion. To protect themselves from such a fate, seeds try to deter predators with antinutrient substances that make us feel sick or resist digestion, or both.[15]

So, if some seeds are safer than others, how do you know which seeds you can eat and which you cannot? Here's a simple rule: if you can eat it raw, like the seeds of strawberries or bananas, it should be OK. If, however, the seed has to be cooked, soaked, fermented, pulverized, or processed before you can eat it, it's not.

Unfortunately the standard American diet is teeming with seeds that require processing, specifically grains. High concentrations of lectins in our diet can create dramatic shifts in our gut flora as they tend to mimic the composition of simple sugars, allowing them to simply pass through the gut lining, damaging or destroying enterocytes along the way.[16]

Once they're through the gut wall, the lectins activate those resident immune cells that start the autoimmune process. Lectins don't travel alone, either; there is evidence that they help transport both dietary and gut-derived pathogens throughout the body,[17] which means that whatever you ate with the grains or legumes is now piggybacking a ride into your circulatory system and causing even more autoimmune reactions. As if that weren't enough, lectins also upset the body's hormone balance and metabolism, interfere with mineral absorption, cause reductions in protein digestibility, and can cause allergic reactions.[18,19,20]

One of the more damaging lectins is gluten, found most abundantly in wheat. It is beyond the scope of this book to go fully into all the dangers of wheat. Dr. William Davis's popular book *Wheat Belly* is a fantastic resource for those who want detailed information on how dangerous the "staff of life" actually is. But for our purposes here, you should be aware that gluten has been associated with numerous negative responses in the body, including acne, fatigue, depression, belly fat, joint pain, acid reflux, and celiac disease.

If that doesn't make you think twice about chowing down on a big, doughy bagel, consider that it not only contains gluten, but also gliaden and wheat germ agglutinin (WGA). Gliaden is a protein that has been shown to increase *zonulin* production.[21] Zonulin regulates the permeability of the space between the enterocytes,[22] increases leaky gut in humans and other animals, and has been found to be a key player in autoimmune disease.[23] In severe cases, some of the gut's enterocyte "doors" may become permanently stuck open. This is sometimes seen in celiac disease and other autoimmune patients who have higher than normal amounts of the protein zonulin in their blood.

And finally, the protein WGA survives cooking and stomach acid and can pass through the gut wall all by itself.[24] It also acts as an adjuvant, meaning that it is particularly good at bringing other things along with it and can amplify your body's response to whatever guests that tag along.

Another extremely damaging lectin is phytohemagglutinin (PHA), the lectin found in red kidney beans. Eat just a handful of raw kidney beans and this lectin can kill you. PHA attacks and disables the enterocytes. Your body reacts to the threat by emptying the entire digestive tract as rapidly and completely as possible to rid itself of the toxic substance. If you survive, you certainly won't ever eat raw kidney beans again.

Soaking, sprouting, fermentation, and cooking can reduce or eliminate lectins in some instances and are traditional techniques used to prepare grains and legumes in many cultures. One notable exception is gluten, which survives all but the longest fermentation and is not broken down by cooking.[25]

The lectin in rice is contained mostly in the bran. If you're going to indulge, skip the brown rice and choose white rice as the bran has been

> Wheat ain't just gluten, any more than southern cooking is just grits.
>
> —Dr. William Davis, *Wheat Belly*

stripped away during processing. Whole grains are neither heart-healthy nor good for you in any way, especially if you are battling HS.

If you eliminate all grains but white rice from your diet and you're still having flare-ups, consider white rice as a trigger. Most of us don't have problems with rice, but some of us do. Rice is extremely high in simple sugars that can aggravate HS symptoms. We'll talk more about the sugar connection in chapter five, *The Hormone Connection*, and chapter eight, *Phase I: The Elimination Diet*.

Don't forget that corn is a grain too—it's not a vegetable, as much as the US Department of Agriculture (USDA) insists that it should be. For some, corn is an HS trigger, which is no surprise considering corn, like other grains, contains lectins. Try to avoid corn on the cob, cornstarch, corn tortillas, corn pasta, and baked goods. Definitely avoid high fructose corn syrup or any product that uses the word "maize." Maize simply means "corn" in Spanish.

> **Watch Out For: All cereal grains,** wheat, rye, barley, oats, rice, corn, sorghum, millet, spelt, triticale and teff, either in whole form or in flours and starches. **All legumes,** especially kidney beans. Also avoid lima beans, fava beans, green beans, soy, peas, and peanuts, either in whole form or in flours and starches, oils and butters.

SAPONINS

Many plants contain varying amounts of a substance called saponins. Saponins are a type of chemical defense against microbes and fungi and are considered *plant steroids*. When we consume them, they can create all sorts of effects, some good but mostly bad.

Saponins penetrate cell membranes, directly into molecules such as proteins. They have the ability to permeate mucous linings (like the gut wall) and stimulate an immune response by increasing antibodies.[26] In a healthy person, this may help fight off infections. In someone with HS and a leaky gut, we don't want extra antibodies floating around—any immune response is basically inflammation.[27] Saponins are used in some vaccines as an adjuvant, i.e., they boost the effectiveness of the vaccine.

Scientists in Canada fed mice quinoa saponins along with the cholera toxin and found an increased presence of the toxin in the blood, liver, spleen, and lungs over control subjects. They concluded that quinoa saponins would make an excellent adjuvant for vaccines because they are very effective at increasing the permeability of mucous membranes.[28]

Other saponins, such as one from Quillaja bark (used to make root beer), have been found to be effective at permeating the mucous lining of the nose and eyes. They also promote the absorption of insulin and antibiotics.[29] Looking at these studies, it is evident that consuming saponins can increase your risk for developing bacterial diseases, allergies, and autoimmunity, since bacteria, proteins, and antigens that would normally stay locked up tight within the intestine are free to join up with the saponins and vacation somewhere fun and new, like your internal organs.

Saponins have even been proven to damage villi,[30] the tiny, finger-like projections on the small intestine that assist in absorbing nutrients from food. When they are damaged, you can quickly become malnourished and sick—even though you may be popping expensive multivitamins. Dietary saponins also reduce iron absorption, which can lead to anemia.

Saponins mimic certain hormones in the body and are believed to be responsible for the pharmacological effects of many Chinese herbs.[31] Luckily, the saponins we eat are weak, usually only creating problems in a dose dependent manner.[32] So, eating quinoa once will not create golf ball-sized holes in your gut. But consume large quantities, and you may flare up. Eating a saponin-rich food like asparagus with one of your trigger foods may increase the response.

Watch Out For: All legumes, including peas, lentils, beans, and peanuts; all soy and soy products; "pseudo grains" such as quinoa, amaranth, and buckwheat; chia and flax seeds; alfalfa and bean sprouts; root beer

Limit: Chestnuts; yuca root (cassava); fenugreek, soapwort, paprika, licorice; asparagus; tomato seeds; garlic, leeks, onions and chives; sugar beets; peppers; eggplant

PHYTATES

Phytic acid, aka phytate, is found in many different plants and is a source of energy for that plant. Unfortunately, human beings lack the digestive enzyme (*phytase*) to break down phytic acid[33] and this can cause all sorts of problems for us. Phytates don't necessarily cause leaky gut in and of themselves, but the nutrient deficiencies they create certainly can. (See sidebar *Nutrient Deficiencies,* page 83.)

Phytates bind to the magnesium, calcium, zinc, and iron in your intestines, making it difficult for your body to absorb those minerals. This is not a good thing. Those minerals are essential to our health. In fact, many experts believe that phytates alone are responsible for the worldwide epidemic of iron-deficiency anemia.[34] Phytates could also account for the magnesium deficiencies we're seeing in modern society, which can contribute to everything from muscle cramping to PMS.[35]

Those of us with HS know how important zinc is—most of us are zinc deficient and are on supplementation. Zinc supplementation has been found to be extremely beneficial in HS patients,[36] so a deficiency is definitely something we want to avoid. Zinc is crucial to the immune system—whether or not we have HS. As for calcium, we all know how important it is for building strong bones and teeth, so anything that robs our bodies of that crucial element is something to be avoided at all costs.

Grains and legumes have high levels of phytates in them, but nuts and seeds contain more. The good news is you can soak, ferment, and sprout virtually all of the phytates out of these foods.[37] These traditional techniques used to be commonplace but have fallen out of favor—perhaps about the same time we started to let machines and corporations make our food. Time is money, after all, and these techniques take time.

Oh, and a bit more good news: certain species of our gut flora (including lactobacilli) can produce phytase, which helps break down phtates. This means that if you have good intestinal flora, you'll have an easier time with foods that contain phytic acid,[38] whether they're traditionally prepared or not.

Watch Out For: Grains, legumes, and raw and roasted nuts and seeds, unless they're soaked, sprouted or fermented. Note: roasted nuts in the store have NOT been soaked first.

ALKALOIDS

What are nightshades? More than any other question, this is the one I'm asked most. Even some registered dietitians and doctors I've spoken to don't know what nightshades are. It's not surprising; they're not on many people's radar. Nightshades don't seem to have anything in common at first glance. But on closer inspection, we learn that they share a similar chemistry.

There are more than two hundred nightshade plants, and most are toxic, deadly even. These include deadly nightshade and jimsonweed. But they also include items that we might find in our grocery carts: potatoes, tomatoes, eggplant, and peppers.

Members of the Solanaceae family, nightshades contain compounds that increase intestinal permeability,[39] which can be extremely aggravating to certain inflammatory and autoimmune conditions like arthritis and HS. In addition to lectins and saponins, nightshades also contain alkaloids and glycoalkaloids (alkaloid and sugars). More than three thousand different types of alkaloids exist in nature, including nicotine, caffeine, morphine, strychnine, and quinine. Alkaloids have pharmacological effects on humans, which means that they can behave like drugs. They also possess the ability to weaken cells and collapse or affect nerve transmission.

Alkaloids are designed to protect the plants from predators (sound familiar?) and contain low-dose poisons concentrated in their leaves, stems, sprouts, and fruits. When these toxins affect the human nervous system, they can cause weakness, confusion, headaches, diarrhea, cramps, and, in severe cases, coma and death.

It's no small coincidence that nightshades—like other leaky gut contributors—happen to be a common HS trigger. But if you are like the majority of HS sufferers, you will find that certain nightshade foods—or perhaps all nightshade foods—are your biggest triggers. You'll be asked to eliminate them from your diet once you get to chapter eight. Chances are, they will be the group of foods you'll least likely be able to reintroduce successfully if you want to keep your HS in remission.[40]

Watch Out For: Potatoes, tomatoes, tomatillos, bell peppers, hot peppers, eggplant, goji berries, tobacco

CASEIN (DAIRY)

According to Sarah Ballantyne, the medical biophysicist behind the blog PaleoMom.com, dairy is *designed* to create a leaky gut:

In newborn infants, a leaky gut is essential so that some components of mother's milk can get into the bloodstream, like hormones and all the antibodies that a mother makes that helps boost her child's immune system. While this is essential for optimal health in babies, it becomes a problem in the adult digestive tract where there are more things present that we don't want to leak into the bloodstream. Drinking milk from a different species seems to make matters worse since the foreign proteins can cause a larger immune response.[41]

Human milk is made for humans. It's designed to signal our hormones that we're ready to grow. It also contains certain antimicrobial compounds that are designed to help establish healthy gut flora in infants. These protective factors are missing in the milk of dairy animals,[42] although scientists are working on developing genetically engineered goats to see if the GMO goat milk will have similar benefits to human milk. Thanks but no thanks.

Dairy contains a hormone called betacellulin, which has the ability to pass through the gut wall, taking fragments of the milk protein casein along with it, and whatever else you've eaten with your meal.[43] That's bad news. Casein, the main protein in milk, also has immune-compromising properties.[44]

Dairy has also proved to be insulinemic, meaning that a lot of insulin gets released when you consume it. Lots of insulin means more insulin-like growth factor 1 (IGF-1). IGF-1 regulates cell growth and development and has insulin-like effects in the human body. Cow milk actually contains large amounts of bioidentical IGF-1, so it's a double whammy. (Cow IGF-1 is identical to human IGF-1, so when we consume it, it acts like our own hormones.) That ends up being especially bad for HS, since elevated insulin levels result in increased growth of the skin around the hair follicles. We'll discuss why this is such a problem for us in chapter five, *The Hormone Connection.*

For susceptible people, dairy causes acne, allergy symptoms, and asthma and has been directly linked to cancer and autoimmune conditions such as arthritis and multiple sclerosis. Insulin, IGF-1, and the elevated levels of estrogen in milk from pregnant cows (the very milk you purchase at the supermarket) has been directly linked to prostrate cancer in men.[45] If that isn't enough, consumption of milk (but not cheese and yogurt) has been shown to bring on early menstruation in girls.[46]

Paleo experts such as Sarah Ballantyne, Loren Cordain, Robb Wolf, and Chris Kresser all suggest the removal of dairy for optimal gut health. I suggest removing it not only for gut health, but also for hormonal stability.

If you do choose to reintroduce dairy after you've done your elimination diet, the best choice is grass-fed, full fat, and raw. Fermented is good too *if* you aren't dealing with yeast issues. If you are able to reintroduce dairy without issue, make sure that you stay away from conventional dairy products. They are homogenized, pasteurized, low- and nonfat, and laden with hormones, pesticides, and antibiotics.[47] Obviously, you'll want to avoid any sweetened dairy products as well.

How will you get your calcium, you ask? It's interesting to note that in order for your body to absorb the calcium in "healthy" lowfat dairy products, it requires fat and magnesium to go along with it. Get your calcium from green leafy vegetables cooked in bacon fat; your bones and teeth will thank you.

Watch Out For: Nonfat or lowfat milk; flavored milk products; pasteurized and homogenized dairy products; cheese, especially processed; frozen yogurt, sweetened yogurt, yogurt in a tube; anything containing "sodium caseinate," "calcium caseinate" and "milk protein" on labels.

NUTRIENT DEFICIENCIES

Lectins, phytates, and saponins block our body from absorbing vital nutrients such as zinc, magnesium, calcium, iron, and copper. Other antinutrients called pyridoxine glucosides, which can be found in grains and legumes, block the absorption of important B vitamins.[70]

All these nutrients are needed to maintain the intestinal barrier and play an important role in all areas of your body. Zinc and vitamin B6 help to produce stomach acid and maintain gut integrity. Vitamin A is essential for building healthy mucosal linings, including those of the intestines.[71] If you are consuming foods with antinutrients in them, you won't be able to absorb these important vitamins and minerals—and your gut won't be able to repair itself.

So did your leaky gut cause your nutrient deficiencies, or did the nutrient deficiencies cause your leaky gut? The answer depends on how long you've been sick and what your diet was like, but in the end it doesn't really matter which came first. The trick is to stop eating the gut-irritating foods so that your intestine can heal—then you'll be able to absorb all those expensive supplements you've been flushing down the toilet all these years. Better yet, you'll be able to absorb all the vitamins and minerals from the food you eat, and you won't need expensive supplements in the first place.

LYSOZYME (EGG WHITES)

It's curious that egg yolk has been vilified, because it's actually the egg white that causes most of the problems.

Egg whites contain lysozyme, an enzyme that is very good at breaking apart the cell membranes of certain bacteria. Sarah Ballantyne has used lysozyme in the lab for this very purpose. "Lysozyme works very quickly, is very resistant to heat, is stable in very acidic environments, and is really a pretty ingenious little enzyme," she says. "It has the ability to form strong complexes with other proteins."

Lysozyme survives cooking and our stomach acid, defies digestion, attaches on to the other proteins in the egg white (and whatever else it comes in contact with, especially bacteria) and sails right through our enterocytes—even in healthy individuals without leaky gut.[48] "The problem is the other proteins that piggyback on lysozyme," explains Ballantyne. Because lysozyme binds to bacteria so well, these are likely to come along for the ride.

"In the case of autoimmune disease, individuals are more sensitive and tend to have exaggerated immune and inflammatory responses to foreign proteins in the circulation," says Ballantyne. "These individuals are also more likely to form auto-antibodies in response to bacterial proteins that may enter into the circulation with lysozyme."

If you are a healthy individual with a healthy gut, you should probably limit your egg intake, but not for the "traditional" reasons of lowering cholesterol or fat intake that may come to mind. If you are suffering from HS or any other autoimmune problem, eggs whites should be off the list entirely while you do your elimination diet. Once your gut flora is well populated with good bacteria, you can experiment with bringing them back into your diet.

We'll return to this topic and examine each of these gut-destroying foods in greater depth in chapter eight, *Phase I: The Elimination Diet.*

The Link Between Drugs and Leaky Gut

Different drugs cause leaky gut for different reasons. There are far too many types of drugs on the market to list them all. I personally found that as I changed my diet and regained my health and vitality, I no longer needed drugs to feel well. When I experienced a symptom that I would have taken drugs for in the past, like bloating or gas, I tried to figure out why I had those symptoms in the first place instead of simply masking them. I was usually able to connect the problem with something I had eaten or come in contact with. Hopefully as you heal, you will no longer need the drugs you may have been dependent on in the past.

As previously mentioned, saponins, lectins and glycoalkaloids are used in some medications. Some drugs, like morphine, simply *are* alkaloids. Saponins are naturally present in a lot of Chinese medicinal herbs. NSAIDs, antibiotics, and birth control pills are all scientifically proven to cause leaky gut because of the way they affect gut flora. Here are some other sources that may surprise you:

ANTACIDS

Antacids contain aluminum hydroxide, or alum. Aluminum is often used as an adjuvant in vaccines, and has been linked to a variety of serious autoimmune and inflammatory conditions.[49] Antacids that contain aluminum hydroxide, as well as some baking powders and antiperspirants, should be avoided. Note: I recently saw alum listed as an ingredient in deli ham. That's right: deli ham. Always check the ingredients.

VACCINES

Vaccines have saved millions of lives on the one hand and have seemingly destroyed lives on the other. Public opinion is heated; people either seem to be big proponents of vaccines, or they are vehemently opposed to them. It's not up to me to try to change your mind, wherever you stand on the debate. That said, vaccines very often contain such adjuvants as lysozyme (eggs), alkaloids, and saponins. Like anything else, weigh the pros and cons of each vaccine you are considering, and make an informed decision for you and your family.

Leaky Gut & Microorganisms

Normally, microorganisms such as various parasites, bacteria, fungi, and mycotoxins move through our intestines and are excreted as waste. However, if we are experiencing constipation, they hang around much longer than normal and can damage the intestinal lining. They can also act on undigested food and produce even more toxic waste, chemicals, and gas. When these toxins enter our bloodstream, they set off our immune responses.

Different microorganisms act differently in our bodies. Viruses tend to be transient, meaning they come and go. Parasites tend to stick around unless you treat them, but can sometimes cause cyclical symptoms (like remission for ten days, followed by a flare-up, followed by remission). Bacteria tend to produce symptoms that are acute, like gas and bloating. And fungi tend to produce more chronic, slowly changing symptoms.[50]

Taking a quality probiotic and healing your gut can help with both constipation and the war against any bad bugs in your tummy. Visit a doctor if you suspect a fungal or parasitic infection.

YEAST OVERGROWTH

As previously discussed, the effects of taking antibiotics or having impaired gut flora can last for years if left untreated. When the bad guys outnumber the good guys, the villains thrive, reproduce, and literally take over.

One of the bad guys that really goes to town is *Candida albicans*. This yeast microorganism normally lives in the intestinal tract of every human, but beneficial bacteria keep it in check. If Candida is allowed to overgrow, it leads to yeast infections, and guess what? Yep, it too can cause leaky gut.

According to the National Candida Center, when Candida overgrowth moves to a more serious stage and becomes a yeast infection, it grows roots or hyphae, which are long, branching cells of a fungus. The hyphae spread the intestinal wall cells (enterocytes) apart so that acidic, harmful microorganisms and macromolecules are able to pass through the openings and enter the circulatory system.[51]

Many things can cause dysbiosis and an overgrowth of Candida;

however, the Center points its finger at the following as the primary causes:

- Prescription hormones (birth control pills and/or hormone replacement therapy)
- Prescription corticosteroids (hydrocortisone)
- Excessive use of antibiotics
- Processed foods contaminated by parasites, fungus, and/or mold
- Increased amounts of refined carbohydrates
- Increased alcohol and caffeine consumption

Essentially anything that causes an upset in our gut flora can lead to a yeast infection. Over-the-counter remedies only treat the immediate symptoms and don't get to the root of the problem. This is why yeast infections tend to reoccur. Wild yeast from foods can also pose a problem for HS and can contribute to leaky gut. We'll discuss yeast in depth in chapters eight and nine.

MYCOTOXINS

Mycotoxins are a toxic byproduct of the fungi kingdom, commonly referred to as mold. The worldwide contamination of food and feed by mycotoxins is a significant problem.[52] Contamination is usually the result of improper storage in wet or humid climates, although food from drier climates can also be affected. The effect of mycotoxins on humans can range anywhere from weight gain and immune suppression to cancer, death, and hallucinations. Both penicillin and LSD are types of mycotoxins.

Foods most commonly contaminated with mycotoxins are cereal grains, peanuts, coffee and cocoa beans, dried fruit, and wine. And milk: if dairy feed is contaminated with mycotoxins, the milk will be too.[53] Also, anything grown in the shade or in wet, humid conditions is susceptible if not processed carefully. Some types of mycotoxins (there are many) can permeate the gut wall, causing leaky gut and autoimmunity.

Lucky for us, most of the foods commonly contaminated with mycotoxins are off of our list anyway. Avoid shade-grown coffee, be very selective when choosing dried fruit and wine, and completely avoid conventional, non-organic dairy sources.

Supplements and Your Gut Health

There are certain supplements that can help improve the integrity and health of your gut, and at the same time, reduce gut permeability. It's a win-win situation. Someone battling HS should consider the following supplements as part of their healing process.

OMEGA-3 FATTY ACIDS

Omega-3 fatty acids, like those found in fish, help to naturally lower inflammation in our bodies. In contrast, omega-6 fats are proinflammatory. Omega-6s come from grain and seeds primarily, and we have way too much of them in our food these days—we get them from our grain-fed meat, vegetable oils, and grains/seeds in our own diets. Eating too many omega-6s instead of omega-3s increases your risk of heart disease and certain forms of cancer; it also makes inflammatory and autoimmune diseases worse.[61] Removing grains and industrial seed oils from your diet will go a long way to reducing your intake.

Unfortunately now that our food animals are passing on omega-6s to us because of what they eat (corn) and we generally don't eat enough fish, I take fish oil to make sure I'm getting enough omega-3s. Grass-fed meat and pastured eggs are also a great source of omega-3, but fish is the best. Cod liver oil has omega-3 in it too, as well as naturally occurring vitamins A and D3, both great for autoimmune conditions.

Believe it or not, flaxseed is not a great source of omega-3s for human beings. Flax contributes a short-chain omega-3 known as alpha-linolenic acid (ALA). This needs to be converted into long-chain omega-3s called eicosapentaenoic acid (EPA) and docosahexaenoic acid (DHA). This process doesn't work very well in the human body and only about 5 to 10 percent of the ALA is actually converted.

Ironically, the more saturated fat you eat, the more efficient the conversion, but many people who take flax tend to avoid saturated fat. Alcohol, diabetes, sugar, aging and high amounts of omega-6 in the diet also lower the conversion rate.

Flax (like soy) also contains xenoestrogens, which mimic our body's own estrogen and can cause hormonal imbalances. If that weren't enough, it also contains antinutrients, which can irritate the gut lining and cause leaky gut in some people.

Instead of taking a precursor to omega-3 that isn't efficiently converted and can actually cause damage, you'll probably find that getting anti-inflammatory omega-3s straight from the source is going to work much better. The ratio of omega-6 to omega-3 fats in our early ancestors was somewhere around 1:1 to 2:1.[62] The average modern American's omega-6 to omega-3 ratio is anywhere from 20:1 to 200:1, depending on their diet.

PROBIOTICS AND PREBIOTICS

It's important to take a quality probiotic supplement if you want to heal your gut and end your HS symptoms. Yogurt, kefir, kimchi, some aged cheeses, raw sauerkraut, kombucha, and brine-cured pickles are all natural sources of probiotics, but they are problematic to anyone with yeast sensitivities. That's nearly everyone who suffers from HS.

So how do you get your probiotics? Through regular probiotic supplements, like lactobacillus, which do not contain yeast. In fact, some strains of beneficial bacteria, like bacillus coagulans, bacillus subtilis, and enterococcus faecalis, are used to combat yeast.

If you are currently on antibiotics, take probiotics at opposite times of the day. If you determine that you are not yeast intolerant (we'll discuss this more in chapters eight and nine), you can also get a product that contains *Saccharomyces boulardii*, beneficial yeast that isn't affected by most antibiotics. *S. boulardii* has been shown to improve leaky gut all by itself, to prevent antibiotic-associated diarrhea, and in some cases, has even worked better than antibiotics alone for parasites.[54,55]

You may have heard of prebiotics and wondered how they differ from probiotics. Probiotics are the microorganisms and prebiotics are their food. If you feed and nourish the good bacteria in your gut, you won't need to replenish them as often.

Prebiotics are primarily found in chicory, bananas, kiwi, onion, and garlic, but smaller amounts can be found in quite a few other fruits and vegetables. Supplements are available but research on prebiotics is still in its infancy. For now, it's probably best to get your prebiotics from natural sources.

> A vitamin is a substance that makes you ill if you don't eat it.
>
> —Albert Szent-Gyorgyi, Nobel Prize in Physiology or Medicine, 1937

VITAMIN A

Vitamin A, also known as retinol, is a fat-soluble vitamin. It's only found in foods that come from animals, so vegetarians and vegans are at increased risk of vitamin A deficiency (among other things).

As discussed, nutrient deficiencies are often the result of a leaky gut— and a leaky gut can't be repaired without certain key nutrients. Vitamin A helps protect our mucous membranes, which includes the lining of our digestive tract. If we're deficient, the integrity of the gut lining can be compromised.

Vitamin A also affects our skin. It causes drying, which affects the texture and appearance of our skin. It also affects cell division and speeds up the exfoliating process; skin cells turn over more often, which usually results in clearer skin, and since sebum and keratin aren't excessively produced when vitamn A levels are sufficient, our pores don't get clogged. Retinol is used in beauty creams because it works wonders on skin conditions—even Accutane is a form of vitamin A. The vitamin has been shown to help virtually every skin condition that responds to exfoliating agents and keratolytics (something that helps counter keratin).

This is because vitamin A regulates keratin production; having low blood retinol levels means your body is going to crank up keratin production, and store it, too. That is what sucks for us—our hair follicles get blocked with keratin, and it causes boils, pimples, zits, bumps, and ingrown hairs, not to mention dry, scaly, and cracked skin. Increasing the amount of vitamin A you take in is very important if you want smooth, healthy, soft skin; we need keratin production, among other things, to be lowered in order to achieve remission.

Before you reach for the supplements, I would encourage you to try to get your vitamin A from natural sources. Vitamin A can be obtained from fruits and vegetables in the form of beta carotene, but just like with the conversion of ALA in flax to DHA, the conversion of beta carotene to retinol in our body isn't perfect. Supplementing with vitamin A pills can be dangerous—retinol gets stored in our body—so getting enough from natural food sources (which you can't overdose on) is important.

Once your gut heals, you'll be able to absorb more vitamin A from the foods you eat. Fermented cod liver oil (also rich in vitamin D) is arguably one of the best natural, bio-available sources of vitamin A you can get, but other good sources include liver, eggs, and butter.

You can also try a natural vitamin A cream to speed up skin cell turnover, although you should be aware that it may cause excessive drying, peeling, or even a sunburn. Keratolytic products, such as salicylic acid, can also be helpful, as they contribute toward the exfoliating process.

VITAMIN C

Vitamin C, or ascorbic acid, helps reduce inflammation and gives your immune system a positive boost. It also helps shut down excessive activation of the immune system to prevent tissue damage, supports antibacterial activity, and interferes with the creation of proinflammatory cytokines.[66] And it protects our immune cells against free radicals and plays a crucial role in the formation of skin.[67]

VITAMIN D3

Cholecalciferol, or vitamin D3 isn't actually a vitamin; it's a pre-hormone. It acts in every cell of our body and influences hormones. It's one of the big players and most of us are deficient.

DISEASES AND DISORDERS

This may be another case of the chicken and the egg: which came first? Inflammation of the intestine causes leaky gut, which causes inflammation of the intestine. This aggravates conditions such as Crohn's disease, celiac disease, IBS and IBD, which in turn opens the door for further autoimmune problems, such as HS. Many medications used to control different diseases can also cause leaky gut, either through gut dysbiosis or other means. Food allergies, which may have been created due to a leaky gut, can also exacerbate the problem.

As you begin to heal, you may find that syndromes and conditions you used to have are suddenly gone, or at the least, very manageable. Making sure you pay attention to every symptom your body relays to you is of the utmost importance.

There are a few reasons for this. First of all, very few of us spend several hours a day in the sun, wearing nothing but a loincloth. When we are in the sun, we slather sunscreen on any exposed skin to "protect" us from skin cancer. Our bodies naturally produce vitamin D3 when exposed to sun, but depending on the pigment of your skin and where you live, you would need to spend a substantial amount of time outside practically naked to make enough on your own.

Second, there are very few natural food sources of vitamin D3. Food products that have it added to them usually use a different form of the hormone: ergocalciferol, or vitamin D2. This form of the hormone isn't fully recognized or assimilated by our bodies, doesn't raise blood levels of vitamin D, and is also linked to cancer.[56]

Third, most of the supplements haven't been suspended in fat. Vitamin D3 is a fat-soluble hormone, meaning that you need to take it with fat in order for your body to absorb it. Supplements suspended in olive oil are especially good; anything that comes in a pill you may as well flush down the toilet (these are usually D2, anyway).

Fourth, those of us that are taking the proper supplements aren't taking enough. Current recommendations for vitamin D3 are 400 IU per day. That is absolutely laughable. I can't tell you how much to take, but I can tell you that I personally take between 5,000 and 10,000 IU a day. Getting a blood test done to see what your vitamin D levels are is a great starting point to see how much you need to take.

Fifth, and probably most important, the high fiber diets we've been told are SO important to our health actually lead to increased elimination of vitamin D3 from our bodies.[57] Researchers postulate that this last factor alone could account for the development of vitamin D3 deficiency in Asian people with normal exposure to light.

This study was done in 1983. The fact that dietary recommendations for fiber have increased since then makes me so mad I could spit. Fiber from fruits and vegetables doesn't have much of an impact, but the fiber found in cereal grains, especially wheat, has been shown to be especially problematic. Feeding wheat bran to "healthy" volunteers caused them to burn through their vitamin D3 reserves at an accelerated rate.[58]

Vitamin D3 is critical in managing insulin resistance and autoimmunity. It regulates and normalizes immune responses.[59] Animal studies have found that certain autoimmune responses can be prevented simply by dosing the animals with high levels of D3 beforehand.[60]

Leaky gut can prevent the absorption of fat-soluble vitamins, so it's not a matter of whether or not you need to take vitamin D3, it's a matter of how soon you can get it into your bloodstream. Make sure you're also getting quality sources of vitamin K2 in your diet, as well. You can find K2 in seafood, grass fed meats, organ meats, and pastured egg yolks.

I suggest taking vitamin D3 first thing in the morning. I have found it interferes with my sleep, otherwise. Try to get out in the sun as much as possible and maintain a light tan, if you can.

ZINC

A lot of people with HS report benefits from supplementing with zinc or from using zinc cream on their boils. Dr. Loren Cordain says that "zinc supplementation (90 mg/day for three months) has been shown to reduce inflammation in HS patients."[63]

A 2007 pilot study combining HS and zinc in France had spectacular results. They found a clinical response in all test subjects, with complete remission in 36 percent of them,[64] at the doses recommended by Cordain.

Another study from France in February 2012 proved the benefits of using zinc supplementation in HS treatment and showed a possible autoimmune connection at the same time. Researchers observed that HS prone skin had "significantly decreased expression of all the innate immunity markers," with lesional HS skin levels being even lower. Three months of zinc treatment resulted in a significant increase in the markers involved in innate immunity,[65] meaning that autoimmune responses were lessened.

Patients were tested using zinc gluconate, the same stuff you can buy for about two bucks a bottle.

MAGNESIUM

Magnesium is essential to our health. It's the fourth most abundant mineral in the body and is needed for more than three hundred biochemical reactions. Besides keeping bones strong, maintaining muscle and nerve function, and supporting a healthy immune system, magnesium helps to regulate blood sugar and blood pressure and can sometimes be used to manage diabetes. It also helps us go to the bathroom; anyone who's been constipated and has taken magnesium can attest to that.

Green leafy vegetables are a great source of magnesium but most of us don't eat enough to get the daily recommended intake. Add this to the fact that antinutrients in grains, legumes and nuts can deplete our bodies of magnesium and it's no wonder why most of us are deficient.

I've found that taking a regular magnesium supplement helps keep me "regular." Since constipation can actually cause leaky gut and is a symptom of it too, being regular is a good thing.

Are We There Yet?

Yes. We're there. All the major players covered regarding leaky gut, anyway. Anything else that causes leaky gut that wasn't covered in this chapter hopefully isn't your problem. If it is, you're going to need more help than I can give you. There are, however, a couple more factors in the equation besides leaky gut that we're going to have to cover in order to put our HS into remission. We'll deal with hormones and stress in the next chapters coming up.

You won't necessarily need to remove everything I mentioned in this chapter from your diet forever, so don't panic. Just drop most of it for thirty to sixty days and you will be able to add a lot of it back in.

We'll be covering what you ARE supposed to eat, which medications are still safe to take, and how you're supposed to go about it all this in the second half of this book, *The HS Autoimmune Protocol.* I started with the depressing stuff, but there is good news:

You can still eat bacon.

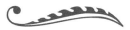

CHAPTER FIVE
The Hormone Connection

*"We're trying to use a thing we don't
understand, to understand ourselves."*
—Meshell Ndegeocello

*I*dentifying your food triggers and healing your gut are very important, but they are only part of the equation. As you might suspect, hormones also play a huge role in HS. Women reading this book are probably nodding their heads because our flare-ups often coincide with our menstrual cycles. But even if you don't menstruate, you're not immune to the power of hormones. If you seem to flare up after you consume sugar, experience stress, or for no apparent reason, the rise and fall of certain hormones, and how they interact, can certainly shed some light on why that is.

There are about two hundred different hormones in our bodies (that we know about), each charged with their own job, and all intricately connected. They exist to create balance and stability within the body. If one hormone is out of whack, it affects all the others and creates a cascade of problems. I won't go into depth about every hormone in the human body, but I will discuss those that come into play during a flare-up. This will help you to achieve remission, and I guarantee you'll be surprised. The hormones to blame are not the ones you think.

Why Do I Flare Up Before My Period?

Women are two to five times more likely to get HS than men, and the average age that HS starts is twenty-three. That means that if you're reading this book, there's a pretty good chance you are a menstruating female.

You may happen to see HS flare-ups right before or during your period due to a combination of hormones, stress, and trigger foods. All autoimmune diseases can be affected by the level of hormones in the system and are therefore sensitive to the changes that occur to hormone levels during menstruation.[1] It's not just people with HS who complain of flare-ups before their period; a quick google search turned up complaints concerning arthritis, asthma, Crohn's disease, thyroid disease, and more.

It's common for women to believe that their HS is caused solely by the hormonal shifts of their periods. But your period *alone* isn't causing the HS. If this were the case, men wouldn't get HS. Men don't have periods and they don't have the same level of hormones in their bodies as women. And yet, men get HS.

If HS were caused by your period, then you would spontaneously go into remission when you hit menopause. That doesn't happen. I have also talked to parents with prepubescent daughters who suffer from HS.

In line with the research I've done, experiments on myself, and the testimony I've received from others, I can only conclude that *sex hormones alone do not cause HS*. If they did, everyone would have it; *everyone* to some degree has estrogen, testosterone, and progesterone coursing through their body, with daily, weekly, monthly, and even *annual* fluctuations of all three. At the very least, if sex hormones were solely responsible, we would see much, much higher rates of HS—it would be commonplace. If you're still in doubt, remember there are menstruating women out there who have managed to put their HS into remission. There are also women who have gone through menopause who are still battling HS.

Clearly, sex hormones are not solely to blame for HS. They do, however, set the stage for certain things to occur, especially when combined with a leaky gut and gut-irritating foods. Let's examine the various hormones that come into play during your monthly cycle, so you can see how they affect your HS.

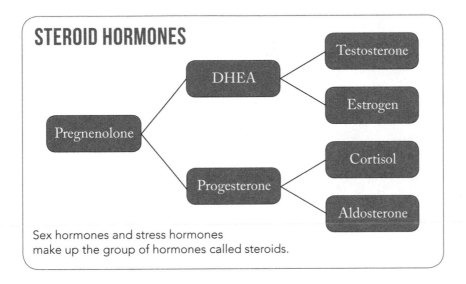

STEROID HORMONES

Pregnenolone → DHEA → Testosterone, Estrogen

Pregnenolone → Progesterone → Cortisol, Aldosterone

Sex hormones and stress hormones
make up the group of hormones called steroids.

The Sex Hormones

Sex hormones—testosterone, estrogen, and progesterone—fall into a group called *steroid hormones*. These hormones are made in the human body from cholesterol. They all start life off as a master hormone known as *pregnenolone*. Depending on the body's needs and current level of balance, pregnenolone is converted (via pathways) into each one of the following hormones on a daily basis.

TESTOSTERONE

Testosterone is an anabolic hormone; that means that it causes the body to grow and develop. Testosterone is a type of androgen. In men, testosterone is responsible for the deepening of the voice, the growth of the beard, and other masculine features. In women, testosterone makes us feel more interested in sex. Our bodies also convert some of it to estrogen.

One of the symptoms of excess testosterone is acne. Testosterone can change the thickness of the skin, affect wound healing, cause changes to the sebaceous (oil) glands, and make hair grow faster and thicker[2]— all things that can affect your HS. Androgens, along with IGF-1, play a major role in clinical acne in both adult men and women.[3] And one study has shown that nearly all HS patients have excess testosterone levels and about half have acne,[4,5] so as we discussed in chapter two, androgen blockers are popular treatments for HS.

I'M A MAN, I DON'T GET PERIODS

Believe it or not, men DO have cyclical surges of hormones. They're just not marked by an obvious event like a period. According to recent studies, not only do men have daily surges of LH and FSH, they also experience seasonal fluctuations of testosterone and estrogen, with testosterone peaking in the spring and waning in the fall.[11,12] Men also make progesterone, which is used for electrolyte balance and to regulate stress hormones.

Testosterone in men varies from hour to hour, with peaks in the morning. Men who track their moods, sexual desire, energy, frustration, and weight throughout the month will see a pattern emerge. Men even go through something called andropause, which is the male equivalent of menopause. Unfortunately, each man's "cycle" is completely unique to him so it can be frustrating to track and is completely individual. A man's cycle may last anywhere from one to six weeks.

Having any of these hormones out of whack could result in more flare-ups than normal. If you suspect a hormone imbalance, consider testing your androgen levels. I also suggest stabilizing your insulin to help balance your other hormones.

ESTROGEN

Estrogen plays a couple different roles when it comes to HS. Normally thought of as the "woman's hormone," estrogen is equally important in men. It is an anabolic hormone and is responsible for the growth of characteristics that we have come to associate with women. It also helps with building bone mass and promotes lung function. In fact, estrogen has more than four hundred roles in the body, some of which affect our skin.

Estrogen makes secretions from the oil glands more fluid and counters the acne-causing effects of testosterone.[6] Essentially, it keeps your pores from getting clogged. Estrogen also promotes glucose availability and uptake into muscle fibers,[7] meaning that it helps you metabolize carbohydrates and sugar. (See section *Why Do I Flare Up Before My Period?*) On the other hand, estrogen suppresses protein metabolism.[8]

Birth control pills that contain estrogen are usually the first treatment prescribed for acne and are often recommended for HS. Medications that contain a combination of estrogen and progesterone are also prescribed. Unfortunately the effects of progesterone on our skin create the perfect environment for HS flare-ups.

PROGESTERONE

Progesterone is also an anabolic steroid hormone and is used to make other hormones, including the stress hormones cortisol and aldosterone, which we will touch on soon. However, progesterone does quite a few things all by itself, some of which can affect our HS.

Progesterone has the opposite effect of estrogen on our skin.[9] It stimulates the production of sebum, a thick oily substance that acts as a natural skin lubricant. For some people, this gives them a healthy, natural glow. For others, it creates an oil slick. As progesterone levels rise, your skin swells and your pores are compressed shut. This makes the sebum build up under the skin's surface and creates the perfect environment for a pimple or boil. At the same time, progesterone raises epidermal growth factor-1 (EGF-1) levels, which stimulates the growth of skin cells.

That's not all. Progesterone also plays an important role in the signaling of insulin release. It's worth noting that people with high progesterone levels are more susceptible to insulin resistance and diabetes. Ever wonder why pregnant women need to be tested for gestational diabetes, something that can only happen when you're pregnant? During pregnancy, progesterone is the dominant hormone; its presence is necessary to ensure that the pregnancy continues. High levels of progesterone give pregnant women that "glow." But it comes at a price. Progesterone promotes the metabolism of protein while it inhibits glucose uptake into cells,[10] which can make you diabetic. After birth, when progesterone levels return to normal, the diabetes spontaneously "disappears."

Progesterone is not normally prescribed as a treatment for HS, as there is no logical, scientific reason for doing so. I have, however, spoken to one poor woman whose doctor tried giving her progesterone supplements to "help" with the HS. Like I said, doctors are getting creative.

> *Science has proven that while your genes control your biology, a rather simple, nondrug formula of nutrient-rich food, targeted supplements to address missing precursors, and lifestyle changes can keep your genes in perpetual 'repair' mode.*
>
> —Sara Gottfried,
> *The Hormone Cure*

Hormone Fluctuations

By now, you should have a pretty good understanding of what sex hormones do. Now, let's find out how monthly hormone fluctuations can result in HS flare-ups that are clustered around your period.

Let's assume that your period is the standard twenty-eight-day cycle. Even if it's off a little from that (or completely irregular), there are some cues that will help you figure out where you are in relation to your hormones.

THE FOLLICULAR PHASE (APPROXIMATELY DAY 1 TO DAY 14)
Day one is the first day of your period, and luteinizing hormone (LH), follicle stimulating hormone (FSH), progesterone, and estrogen are at their lowest levels. Testosterone remains constant throughout the cycle, so that means testosterone is the dominant hormone on day one. But soon after bleeding starts, the ovaries start to excrete estrogen. The rising levels of estrogen trigger the growth of the uterine lining. During the latter part of the follicular phase, estrogen becomes the dominant hormone. And since it promotes glucose metabolism, you may find that you are able to consume sugar or a trigger food without penalty during this time.

MID-CYCLE: OVULATION
As ovulation approaches, estrogen levels continue to rise, as do LH and FSH, the hormones responsible for ovulation. When the follicles in the ovary start to mature, the ovaries secret a surge of progesterone in addition to the estrogen. At this time, you may flare up. Pay special attention to the pores on your nose and any oil on your skin: when your progesterone surges, your pores will look minimized and your face and hair may become oily. Since progesterone inhibits glucose metabolism and signals insulin release, if you eat sugar or a trigger food during this time, you may experience inflammation or a flare-up.

THE LUTEAL PHASE (APPROXIMATELY DAY 15 TO DAY 28)
The luteal phase lasts about fourteen days, approximately the last half of your cycle. Progesterone levels continue to increase and it becomes the dominant hormone during the second half of your cycle. If you eat sugar or a trigger food during this time, you may flare up but it won't

necessarily be as bad as what's coming in a week or two.

A few days before the end of your cycle, both estrogen and progesterone levels dramatically drop off (if you haven't gotten pregnant). This triggers your period and can also cause fluid retention. (This is the aldosterone talking.) As bleeding approaches, testosterone is once again the dominant hormone. **This is the magical time when most of us flare up.** This "danger zone" can be anywhere from a week before your period until several days after it starts. Avoid all sugar and trigger foods during this time. (Cravings will be at their strongest during this phase, which is why many of us give in and indulge ... and flare up.)

The Stress Hormones

CORTISOL

You've probably heard of cortisol—it's the hormone that gets released when we're under stress. It's made from progesterone and is quite necessary. However, prolonged stress (something our bodies were not designed to handle) causes the body to steal pregnenolone from other pathways in order to fill the demand for extra cortisol. This results in all kinds of hormonal imbalances. Part of the problem is that symptoms appear slowly and gradually; you may be all kinds of messed up by the time you realize your cortisol levels are out of whack.

High levels of cortisol screw up the normal functioning of your immune system and lower your ability to prevent infection and disease. They can hinder the functioning of the thyroid gland, cause high blood pressure, hyperglycemia, and even make you gain weight—especially around your midsection.

Cortisol can also contribute to changes in your skin. Acne, increased sensitivity, and purple-colored stretch marks have been reported as a result. It doesn't stop there; elevated cortisol can also manifest as depression, paranoia, anxiety. And it can throw off a women's menstrual cycle and kill libido in both men and women.

ALDOSTERONE

This important hormone is also made from progesterone. It is secreted by the adrenal glands and helps regulate the salt and water balance in your body. Like insulin regulates blood sugar, aldosterone regulates electrolytes.

If you have high levels of aldosterone, you will typically have high blood pressure that doesn't respond to normal medication. You may also have weakness, headaches, fatigue, tingling, numbness, and temporary paralysis. Aldosterone secretion can be temporarily elevated due to sodium deficiency and stress. (On the flipside, stress can also steal progesterone that would have normally been used to make aldosterone to make cortisol instead. This is called *the cortisol steal*.)

A lack of aldosterone can affect our skin. Receptors for the hormone are found in skin cells, sweat, and sebaceous glands. Aldosterone receptors are also found in the hair follicles[13] and cause us to excrete excess sodium when we sweat. It's aldosterone's job to reabsorb sodium within the body, so that we always have enough to maintain electrolyte balance. When we have too much sodium in our diet, aldosterone production is decreased and sodium excretion can become defective.[14] This can actually increase sweating. Salt can harden the sebum in these glands, causing it to stick in your pores and create the conditions for a flare-up.

POSTMENOPAUSAL WOMEN AND PREPUBESCENT GIRLS

It takes a while for our guts to get leaky and our bodies to become insulin resistant. That's why hidradenitis suppurativa doesn't usually show up until we're in our early twenties. But there are exceptions, including some young, prepubescent girls who are badly afflicted. I would guess that in these cases, insulin, testosterone, a leaky gut, and the bad fortune to have the autoimmune gene passed on to them are probably the major players. Following a low-glycemic ancestral diet and removing major trigger foods will likely help more than anything else.

Some women experience some relief from their HS once they hit menopause. But many women do not. Studies have found that during the transition from premenopause to postmenopause, SHBG levels begin to increase in insulin-sensitive women, but decrease in insulin-resistant women.[15] This would mean that insulin-resistant postmenopausal women have more free testosterone and less estrogen—a bad combination for HS. Again, a low-glycemic ancestral diet will give these women the best chance at putting their HS into remission.

SEX HORMONE BINDING GLOBULIN (SHBG)

Steroid hormones are fat soluble and can't move around easily in our watery blood. This is where sex hormone binding globulin (SHBG) comes in. SHBG is a special protein carrier that binds to sex hormones, specifically testosterone and estrogen. SHBG likes testosterone the best and will bind to as much of it as it can. Unfortunately once SHBG has bound to testosterone, the hormone becomes "biologically unavailable." That means it's out of commission and can't be used to supercharge our sex lives, muscles, brains, and all the other awesome things we've come to associate with testosterone.

So where does this SHBG come from? It is mostly made in the liver and gets released into the bloodstream, where it goes about sucking up testosterone like a vacuum cleaner. Only about 2 percent of the testosterone in our bodies is leftover, free to do its job. But that amount can fluctuate.

If SHBG levels become too low, there is more free testosterone floating around in our bloodstream. When this happens, our bodies might convert that extra testosterone to estrogen in an attempt to bring SHBG levels back up. But that doesn't always happen. It really depends on a lot of other variables going on inside your body. But suffice it to say that in the presence of too much testosterone we pretty much become sex-crazed maniacs covered in acne and boils, with hair growing or falling out all over the place.

So how do you prevent your SHBG levels from going too low? To answer that question, we have to look at what decreases SHBG production in the first place: insulin, growth hormone, IGF-1, and androgens (testosterone). SHBG is also significantly decreased in people who are insulin resistant.[16] Anything that increases androgen levels—like anabolic steroids, PCOS, hypothyroidism, diabetes, obesity, and Cushings syndrome—will further lower the amount of SHBG in the blood. Other factors, such as pro-inflammatory cytokines, can also decrease SHBG.[17] Studies have shown that patients suffering from low-grade chronic inflammatory diseases like HS have low blood levels of SHBG.[18] By default, that means that excess testosterone is playing a part in the condition, but that *excess insulin is really the instigator.*

On the flip side, any estrogenic state (when levels of estrogen are high) causes an increase in SHBG. Birth control pills, pregnancy, hyperthyroidism, cirrhosis, anorexia nervosa, and certain drugs all cause high levels of estrogen. This is why HS and other skin-related problems like acne go into remission during these times. Thyroid hormones also cause SHBG to increase,[19] putting the person in an estrogenic state and making it difficult to lose weight.

It really is a delicate balance. You don't want your SHBG to be too low or too high. When SHBG levels are high, we may find that we have a testosterone deficiency, which can lead to loss of libido, anxiety, fatigue, increased abdominal fat, and hair loss. We can also end up with estrogen dominance, which will in turn, affect our progesterone levels.

So what does this mean for us? Testosterone, estrogen, progesterone, and all of our other hormones play very important roles in our skin. If we have an excess of one, or a deficiency in another, it is going to cause certain symptoms. If we can normalize our levels of SHBG, eventually our other hormones should also normalize. So, how do you do that? Simple. The exact same way you correct *all* the other hormones we've discussed so far. You correct SHBG levels by normalizing insulin production.

Respect Insulin and Find Balance

Believe it or not, *insulin is behind all the hormonal problems associated with HS.* That's right: insulin, that delicately tuned instrument we've been abusing and ignoring all these years on the standard American diet (SAD). In *The Primal Blueprint*, Mark Sisson does a fantastic job explaining the intricacies of insulin. I realized I had a problem with insulin after reading his book and was thrilled to find out that by following an ancestral diet I could corrected my insulin problem. What's more, by correcting your insulin, you also correct other hormonal problems.

So here's the scoop on insulin: its been around since the beginning of human evolution. In fact, it is so old that other hormones in our body were actually *built upon* it. Simply put, there is not a hormone in the body that insulin doesn't affect, if not directly *control.*[20] We don't respect it nearly enough.

We *think* it's biggest job is to control our blood sugar, but it turns out insulin's a little higher in the pecking order than previously assumed. Insulin's main agendas are regulating lifespan and storing nutrients.[21] It is the mob boss controlling the whole warehouse.

We have to get our insulin levels down if we have any chance of getting our other hormones in line and going into remission. In order to fully understand insulin, we need to understand what happens in our bodies when we eat. We need to understand sugar.

SUGAR

Sugar depresses our immune systems by competing with vitamin C for valuable white blood cells, so we get sick more often when we eat it. It's addictive and causes horrible cravings and mood swings. It makes us fat and tired. As bad as all that is, the *worst* thing sugar does to us is something we can't see or feel: it ages us.

You may think that your diet is already relatively free of sugar, but unless you are on a ketogenic (carb-free) diet, I can assure you it's not. When we eat, our digestive system breaks down our food so it can be used as fuel. Any protein we eat gets turned into amino acids. Fats get broken down into fatty acids. And carbohydrates into glucose. Glucose is sugar.

Whole grain bread, carrots, rice, gummy bears, spinach, chocolate cake, or juice, it doesn't matter—your body converts any carbohydrate in your food to glucose and releases insulin to deal with the load. When you take this into account, it's easy to see that your diet may actually be higher in sugar than you might think

Cutting excess sugar out of your life immediately is the best thing you can do for your HS. I'm not saying you can never eat oranges again, but the fat-free Twizzlers have got to go. By the time you complete this book, you will have the tools you need to figure out when you can cheat with sugar, what types of sugar you can tolerate, and what role sugar is playing in your condition.

Once you begin an ancestral diet, you'll find that all sugar and most carbohydrates you're used to eating are off the table. (You'll be getting all the fiber you need from green leafy vegetables and berries and all the energy you need from whole, unprocessed foods instead of grains and legumes, so don't worry.)

I understand that it is almost impossible to avoid sugar for the rest of your life. As you cut sugar out, you will begin to crave it less and less. But beware: when you do indulge, you may find it harder to say no the next time, and the time after that. Our ancestors lived in a world where sugar was scarce. As a result, we are hardwired to eat as much of it as we possibly can, whenever and wherever we see it.

In a sense, sugar is an addictive drug. It changes your brain chemistry. It affects your body in negative ways. It causes inflammation. It can make your HS flare up—even if you are in remission. Plus, if you are still having flare-ups, eating sugar will make them worse.

By eating insulin producing foods, we're shortening how long we live. Keep this in mind when you make your food choices. It may be tempting to eat bucket loads of fruit, cheat with donuts, use artificial sweeteners, drink diet soda, anything to keep that sweet taste in your system. Your brain will be screaming for it during the first few weeks, so it will be hard to resist. But after about twenty-one days, those cravings will subside. Your taste buds will actually change, and you'll find that you begin to crave different foods.

Eventually, you will find the amount of natural sugars that your body can tolerate, and you'll discover the cycles in your body that explain why you experience inflammation from a small amount of sugar one week— yet experience nothing the following week.

Pay special attention to foods containing fructose. Food companies tell us it's safe for diabetics, it doesn't cause blood sugar spikes and dips like regular sugar, and because it is fruit sugar, it's "natural" and "safe." None of this is true.

Fructose acts like poison in our bodies and is toxic in large doses. Nature has provided us with the antidote to that poison. It's called fiber. Anywhere fructose is found in nature—in apples, berries, kiwi, etc.—it will be accompanied by fiber. The problem is that we're just too smart for our own good, and we've managed to separate the two.

Fructose intake has increased dramatically since human beings were hunter-gatherers, outpacing the capacity of human evolution to make the necessary adaptations.[22] Fructose is messing us up in all sorts of ways. The fruits and vegetables we consume today have been selectively bred for higher amounts of sugar, and high-fructose corn syrup, a highly concentrated version of it, is added to practically everything in the supermarket—even to things like vitamin supplements.

There's a condition called fructose malabsorption. If you get gassy, bloated, depressed, and experience acne, you may want to look into it. As you make lifestyle changes, be aware that fructose affects insulin and has been directly linked to inflammation, pro-inflammatory cytokine production, and metabolic syndrome, especially when magnesium deficiency is a factor.[23,24]

A high-fructose diet also leads to elevated cortisol, the major stress hormone we discussed earlier.[25] Fructose also enhances salt absorption, which can give you high blood pressure[26] and aggravate your HS. These two things increase the amount of progesterone our body needs to produce. We don't want elevated levels of progesterone in our system.

I could write an entire book on the dangers of sugar. Instead, I'll keep it short and end with a warning: when I say sugar, I don't just mean fructose, high fructose corn syrup, or white sugar. I don't care if it's natural, organic, raw, unprocessed, handpicked, shade-grown, made from fruit, danced around, or was prayed over before it was harvested. Sugar is sugar.

SUGAR AND INFLAMMATION

When we eat—no matter what we eat—we produce something called free radicals. Free radicals are a normal part of metabolism, and they're usually balanced out by the antioxidants in our food. However, when the amount of free radicals outweighs the antioxidants, it causes problems.

Free radicals play an important role in metabolism, but they are also powerful signals for inflammation and they stimulate the production of pro-inflammatory cytokines.[27] Sugar (even in the form of complex carbohydrates) is associated with increased production of free radicals and pro-inflammatory cytokines.[28]

High-carb diets cause inflammation—even in healthy people. If you're overweight or have metabolic syndrome, this effect is going to be exaggerated: **inflammation is directly proportional to insulin sensitivity.**[29]

Insulin Resistance

Every time you eat carbs, your body creates glucose. At the same time, your body needs to produce and release insulin to deal with that glucose load, which causes inflammation.

Insulin is your body's only defense against too much sugar and it is designed to work best with small, sporadic amounts. Insulin gets released from your pancreas when glucose is detected in the blood. It shuttles that glucose to virtually every cell in your body so that it may be used for energy, or stored for later.

When we've got too much sugar in our blood over a long period of time, the resulting inflammation makes our cells less sensitive to insulin. The pancreas detects that we've still got lots of glucose in our blood, so it releases even more insulin to deal with it. The new insulin can't do its job either, so the cycle repeats over and over. Even though we have lots of sugar in our blood, it isn't getting to our cells, so we're tired and hungry all the time. We have become insulin resistant.

If you are insulin resistant but have not yet developed type-2 diabetes, the doctor may have told you that you have *metabolic syndrome, syndrome X*, or *pre-diabetes*. There are many diseases and conditions associated with metabolic syndrome, including type-2 diabetes, high blood pressure, heart disease, bad cholesterol, gout, hypoglycemia, obesity, cancer, PCOS, and acne.[30]

Many people with HS suffer from at least one of these things. There is a reason that many people think their HS is connected to being overweight. The sad truth is that everything is connected—just not in the way they think.

High levels of insulin cause tremendous problems for us. First of all, there is evidence that *insulin itself causes inflammation*.[31] So, we've got inflammation from the glucose and inflammation from the insulin. We're tired all the time because our cells aren't getting the energy they need, and we're constantly hungry for sugar because our body thinks it's starving. Our bodies are flooded with pro-inflammatory cytokines, which are responding to foreign proteins in our blood and setting off immune responses. Here's the real kicker though: **elevated insulin is directly responsible for increased follicular skin growth.[32] This is a very bad thing for those of us with HS.**

When a boil or a pimple develops, a couple things happen: the skin around the hair follicle speeds up its growth, oil production increases, and the cells in the follicle clump together and plug the follicle. (This is called *follicular occlusion* and is a factor in *all* cases of HS. See page 22.) This is about the time it starts to get painful and we notice it.

The trick is to normalize your insulin levels and regain insulin sensitivity by reducing the amount of sugar and carbohydrates you eat. If you do this, the skin around your hair follicles should grow normally and you will have solved one piece of the puzzle.

So, insulin makes us insulin resistant, causes inflammation, and provides the perfect conditions for HS flares. But we're forgetting the big news: insulin also directly controls all our other hormones.

INSULIN AND THE OTHER HORMONES

We possess only *one* hormone to lower blood sugar: insulin. On the flip side, we have four different hormones that can *raise* blood sugar: cortisone, growth hormone, epinephrine, and glucagon.[33] After you've been insulin resistant for a while, your pancreas will start to overcompensate and produce even more insulin, which will effectively lower your blood sugar. Then, all four of those other hormones are going to pour into your system in order to raise your sugar back up.

Let's play *The Six Degrees of Kevin Bacon* and see if we can't bring this back to one of the hormones that your doctor wants to treat. Keep in mind there are hundreds of different pathways this process could take, but we'll keep it to hormones we're all familiar with.

- **Insulin** released
- Insulin lowers blood sugar
- **Cortisol** released in response
- Cortisol raises blood sugar, creates inflammation
- Increased demands for cortisol raise **progesterone** levels
- **Pregnenolone** stolen to make extra progesterone
- Not enough pregnenolone to make **DHEA**
- Congrats! You have an **estrogen/progesterone** imbalance
- And excess **testosterone**!

Every hormone in our body can be linked back to insulin—much the same way that charming movie star can be traced back to everyone else in the entertainment world.[34]

Lucky for you, the ancestral diets listed in this book will improve your insulin metabolism naturally.[35] There is no need for medication. Once you've become insulin sensitive again, all your other hormones should eventually fall into place. **Insulin really is the key to this whole mess.**

There are some people out there who don't have metabolic syndrome or insulin resistance, but still have HS or other autoimmune conditions. The truth is: elevated levels of insulin from a standard American diet may be making the HS worse than it would be otherwise. It may just come down to too much fruit, the occasional potato, and thinking that hummus and chips are the ultimate snack.

If you do further research into this topic, you may learn about certain foods like lean meats that cause insulin to be released. You may start to freak out that you can't eat anything. Relax—*insulin is a necessary hormone.* We don't want to abolish it altogether, we just want to make sure it's working properly and minimize the impact that too much of it has on our health. We also want to start showing our respect to the boss, so he can get back to bigger issues and leave the driving to someone else. We'll learn how to do that in chapter nine, *Phase II: Reintroduction and Designing Your Personal Ancestral Diet.*

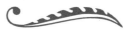

Takeaway Points:
1. Insulin and insulin resistance play a *big* role in HS flares and acne.
2. High progesterone sets the stage for insulin resistance and creates the perfect skin conditions for HS to appear.
3. Insulin resistance causes lower levels of SHBG, which in turn results in more free testosterone in your blood.
4. Testosterone picks up where progesterone leaves off and plays a role in HS flares and acne.
5. When one of your hormones is out of whack, your body, in order to maintain balance, will steal the building blocks for one hormone and turn them into another. This can result in some undesirable side effects.
6. You can correct this whole mess by correcting your insulin levels.

CHAPTER SIX

Wound Care

Our scars tell stories. Sometimes they're stark tales of life-threatening catastrophes, but more often they're just footnotes to the ordinary but bloody detours that befall us on the roadways of life.
—Dana Jennings, *The New York Times*

According to WebMD.com—a medical reference website that has replaced doctors for some people—an abscess is a tender mass, generally surrounded by a colored area from pink to dark red. These masses are easy to feel by touching them. The center is filled with pus and debris. Abscesses can show up anywhere, but when the inflammation is around a hair follicle or oil gland, it's called a boil. If several boils appear in a group, it is a more serious infection called a *carbuncle*.[2]

These abscesses, boils, and carbuncles are what people with HS are trying to get rid of. Since traditional remedies don't work to stop the boils from reoccurring, HS patients will often sabotage their healing by trying all kinds of wacky solutions, creams, poultices, or remedies. Medical literature tells us that these boils should completely resolve and heal within twelve days.[3] But that's often not the case. As

> The average HS patient in secondary care suffers an average of 4.8 boils a month and continues to have an active disease for twenty years after it starts.[1]

many as one-third of all HS boils remain blind, meaning that they fail to come to a head, burst, and discharge the pus. In mild cases, boils remain painful for about two to three days. But on average, boils stay tender for about a week.[4] They take weeks after that to fully subside and resolve. I have personally had HS boils that have taken weeks to come to a head, months to heal, and years for the scars to fade. Often, I would have a second boil appear in the exact same place as one prior, negating all the healing my body had previously done.

To Lance or Not To Lance?

As you get your immune system squared away, your insulin and inflammation in check, and your gut healthy, your flare-ups will become fewer and farther between. Until then, the question remains: How to deal with flare-ups? There are so many private ways to answer this question. Some people can't take the pain anymore and squeeze. They let the lesion scab over, and then squeeze it again. The process can take days and leaves one hell of a scar. It doesn't matter; HS sufferers will do anything it takes to alleviate the pressure and the pain.

Some people prick the lesions with sterilized pins when the pain gets too much to bear. Some go to the doctor and have them lanced. You would think the latter would be the safest solution, but from what I've heard from others this can result in boils that just don't heal. Ever.

"Unfortunately the treatments most commonly used today are the least effective and can be positively harmful," writes Dr. von der Werth. "Incising a ... boil is only going to make matters worse and should be avoided."

As you'll remember from the Surgery section in chapter two, cutting out an existing flare-up and closing the resulting wound is the wrong thing to do, as there is a very high rate of (often immediate) recurrence in such cases. Approximately an 80 percent chance of recurrence.[5] I do not like those odds.

I tried different remedies, including just leaving the boil alone to see what would happen, applying turmeric at different stages, and trying out different antibacterial washes, lotions, and creams. I didn't go to the doctor to have them drained—I was too afraid of the pain.

I know that if you suffer from HS, you've developed a private ritual for taking care of flare-ups when they happen and have likely found *something* that works—and other things that don't. As you're reading, keep in mind that some home remedies are safer than others. If you lance the boils yourself, you are opening yourself up to infection, which could have dire consequences. (On an up note, as you begin healing from the inside, you will reach a stage where the boils no longer need to be drained.)

The method you use to care for your flare-ups is quite dependent on what stage the boil is in—and what stage of HS *you* are in. Any home lancing treatments mentioned in this book pertain to people with mild symptoms. If you have a lesion anywhere near the size of a golf ball, you need to have a professional look at it.

Whether or not the boil is lanced, popped, or just left to run its course, at the end of the day, you need to avoid infection. The pain of an infected boil is excruciating. Steps to avoid infection should be taken with each and every flare-up. Remember, we are dealing with wounds here.

Modern medicine has failed us in many aspects, but hygienic innovations are not included in those failures. If you're able, I suggest seeking out a wound care specialist or a nurse for tips. Even researching basic first aid can give you an idea of how to take care of flare-ups.

If you *must* take measures into your own hands, do practice proper sanitation and refer to the sidebar on the next page, *Draining a Boil*. Note that some HS boils never come to a head. I found that keeping them moist with repeated soakings or wet warm compresses slowed the healing process. I opted instead for a dry, hot compress and kept my wounds as clean and dry as possible. Try a Magic Bag (one of those microwavable hot-cold compresses that usually have beans of some sort in them) and apply over your clothing. The heat is nice and will help with the pain. If you prefer damp heat, you can make a warm compress by soaking a washcloth in hot water, wringing out the excess, and applying to your skin.

Keep in mind that even if a boil has ruptured, it won't heal and the pain will continue if there is even the slightest amount of pus still left inside. Only once the pus is fully drained will the pain cease and the healing begin. If you still experience pain from a rupture that has scabbed over, using wet, warm compresses in this case is a good idea. You'll unfortunately need to fully soften and gently remove the scab in order for the rest of the pus to drain. Be careful, and make sure you sterilize anything you use. Removing scabs can invite infection and scarring.

DRAINING A BOIL

Basic instructions found online for treatment of a boil can help a great deal. I found that following them, with some key changes, helped prevent infection and speed up healing. You will need to work with your doctor or healthcare provider and use your common sense to find an exact procedure that works for you.

According to WebMD, this is the procedure for home treatment of a boil or abscess.

1. Apply warm compresses for thirty minutes, four times a day. This will help to decrease pain and help draw the pus to the surface.
2. Do not attempt to drain the boil by pressing on it, as this can push the infected material into deeper tissues.
3. Once the boil comes to a head, it will burst with repeated soakings. This usually occurs within ten days.
4. When it starts draining, wash with an antibacterial or antimicrobial cleanser, apply medicated ointment and a clean bandage.
5. Wash two to three times a day and use warm compresses until the wound heals.
6. Do not pop the boil with a needle. This can cause or spread infection.
7. If the boil turns red or looks infected, contact your doctor. This also applies if you have a fever over 101.5 degrees Fahrenheit or have red streaks going away from the boil.
8. Go to the emergency room if you have a fever above 102 degrees or have tender lymph nodes.

The Bottom Line

In order for a boil that has come to a head to go away, the following things need to happen: **All of the pus needs to be drained. All of it. And it has to remain free from infection.**

Also, boils heal faster if you treat them the same way as any other open wound. Disinfect it, keep it clean, and let it heal. Don't pick at it and don't put strange things on it, unless you want to tax your immune system even further.

WENDY'S STORY

Self-lancing was so hard to work up the guts to do, but when the pain got really bad it had to be done. I was low tech: get a chair, cover it with a clean towel, get my folding mirror, and other supplies in place. Undress below waist, get in position, heat needle over a flame, clean it with hydrogen peroxide, use mirror to see what I was doing, and firmly guide the tip of the needle as deep as I could stand into the angriest, most pus-filled looking area. Sometimes I was lucky and there was only one that needed lancing, but I've done four at one time during one particularly agonizing flare.

I got a lot of experience in loud, creative F-bombery, that's for sure.

Thankfully, I was usually successful on the first try and the boil would immediately yield pus and blood. I'd blot with sterile gauze as needed, then squeeze gently until I couldn't see any more pus. After things stopped oozing, I'd again blot with new gauze then apply antibiotic ointment, reapplying as necessary a few times a day. Since I could see no way to apply any sort of bandage in that location, I basically tried to keep wounds slathered in antibiotic ointment. As can be imagined, urinating in the days immediately after lancing was extremely unpleasant. I always kept a box of hypoallergenic personal wipes, sterile gauze, and antibiotic ointment right by the toilet so that after I used it I could make sure everything was clean, check if more drainage was needed, and re-apply the ointment.

Overall, I think I was both cursed but still fortunate in the location and size of my HS boils. Nobody but me or my gynecologist could ever see them. The location of the boils was incredibly painful, but they were small and I think their location helped promote wound healing. The inner labia tissues naturally keep themselves moist and well protected. After I lanced and followed the above protocols, I don't ever remember a wound becoming infected.

Wendy, 43
Southeastern Florida

PREVENTING INFECTIONS

The boil itself is actually an infection underneath your skin, but you'll need to make sure that it doesn't become further infected once the skin breaks. At that point, you are vulnerable to anything that broken skin comes into contact with, so you'll need to minimize exposure.

Applying lotions and potions is not recommended. With the exception of sterilization solutions, if you wouldn't eat it, you shouldn't put it on broken skin. Use your common sense on this one.

Pay attention to any fever and redness. If you experience a fever of 101.5 degrees or higher, have red streaks radiating out from the boil, or have tender lymph nodes, you need to get to the doctor immediately.

In my twenty years of suffering from HS, I only got an infected abscess once. Here's what I did to prevent infections:

- Once the boil came to a head and popped, I stopped putting wacky things on it. I made sure it was covered, clean, and dry. Then I just let it heal.
- I washed any clothes, underwear, and bed sheets that had come in contact with my skin in hot water. I also used a dryer to further sterilize them.
- I covered the clean wounds with a padded bandage for at least the first day and night after they started to drain. I found that if I used rubbing alcohol to clean the boil and the surrounding area and let it dry, the bandage would not come off for days. I changed the bandage and cleaned the wound as needed, depending on the amount of drainage or blood. The longer I kept it clean and covered, the faster it healed.
- Once the boil had completely drained and was now just a regular wound, I kept it clean and dry and didn't pick at it.

Hibiclens, an antimicrobial wash used by surgeons, is good for fighting infection. So are Hibistat germicidal hand wipes. Neither do anything to prevent a flare-up, but if one does happen, these items are handy for hastening the healing process. The wipes also help prevent ingrown hairs after shaving. They're also good for treating zits, cystic acne, or clogged pores. Since the wipes are pretty pricey, I suggest cutting one into quarters and storing the pieces in a sealable sandwich bag to use as needed. When money gets tight, regular old alcohol wipes from a first aid kit do the job, but they tend to sting a lot more.

Effective Home Remedies

If you choose to deal with HS flare-ups at home, there are a few things you can do. The following suggestions are not cures for HS, but they can make dealing with flare-ups a little easier.

SHOWER LESS OFTEN

Most of us shower way too often. If you think about the access early modern man would have had to water, what we do today doesn't make sense. We hop into tubs filled with scalding hot water; strip all of the natural oils from our skin, scalp, and hair; spend money on soaps and shampoos that further strip our skin; and then spend hundreds of dollars each year buying products that promise to help replenish the moisture we've lost.

When I lowered the temperature of my showers and committed to showering less often, I had a wonderful surprise. Not only was my hair softer, thicker, and fuller, I no longer needed moisturizer, conditioner, or dandruff shampoo. The changes in my skin were amazing. I didn't smell from bathing less, either; something I had feared when I first tried this experiment. The changes in my diet helped with that. (Once you adopt an ancestral diet, you may find that you no longer need deodorant. This is a very common side effect of "eating clean.")

It was at this time that I had also changed my diet, so I was also experiencing a drastic reduction in the number and severity of HS flare-ups. I found that washing the boils gently with an antibacterial wash sped up healing and prevented infection, but also found that if I washed too often, the healing would slow down.

If, at the very least, you can lower the temperature of your showers, you should see some improvement in your skin. While you are still damp, you can rub coconut oil gently onto your skin. It should be the only moisturizer you need.

If you're showering with a harsh antibacterial wash before your boils come to a head, or as a means of prevention, I've got news for you: it doesn't work. The infection is inside your body, under the skin. These antibacterial washes don't penetrate layers of skin, so they are ineffective as a means of prevention.

I also don't recommend using these washes all over your body. They will unnecessarily strip the oil from your skin in unaffected areas and create dryness. They'll also affect your skin flora and may promote the overgrowth of bad bacteria, which can result in more infection.

Being kind to your skin won't prevent HS, but it may help with healing and scarring. If you are ever in doubt about what methods you should use to treat an open wound on your body, contact your doctor or ask a nurse. They may not know how to prevent HS, but they can help you prevent infection.

DRINK SPEARMINT TEA

Spearmint tea has been shown to have significant anti-androgen effects and can be beneficial when excess testosterone is an issue.[7] A 2010 study found that drinking an infusion of spearmint leaves twice a day for a month can significantly lower free and total testosterone levels while increasing levels of luteinizing hormone and follicle stimulating hormone.[8] The original study in 2007 showed the same results when women drank the tea twice a day for five days during the follicular phase of their menstrual cycles.[9] If you suspect that your HS is aggravated by excess testosterone, drinking spearmint tea may be just as effective as taking a pharmaceutical drug—without the unwanted side effects.

TAKE ZINC

Taking 90 mg of zinc each day helps to reduce inflammation in HS patients.[10,11] This should reduce the size, duration, and pain level of any boil you happen to get. Most of us are zinc deficient, so the fact that too much zinc can block copper (which we've got in spades) won't come into play for quite some time. Though 90 mg a day is a pretty high dose, it seems to be safe and effective for HS.

I also noticed beneficial effects when I applied zinc cream externally, in the form of good old-fashioned diaper cream. Inflammation seemed to be reduced. It felt nice and was soothing, so I considered it a win. Keep in mind that while *zinc gluconate* has been scientifically proven to help reduce inflammation when taken internally,[12] there have been no official studies using zinc *cream* to reduce the size or duration of a boil. Also, you are not supposed to put zinc cream on a gaping wound—there's even a warning on the back of the tube. Once that boil comes to a head and breaks open, you will need to employ standard wound care.

APPLY MANUKA HONEY

Honey has been used for centuries for natural wound healing. Advocates claim it works for everything from sun burns to leg ulcers. Many HS sufferers use manuka honey on their boils.

Honey won't get rid of a boil, make it smaller, or make the pain any less. However, once the boil has come to a head and has opened up, raw honey may help speed healing and avoid infection.

Part of what gives raw honey its antibacterial properties is an enzyme called glucose oxidase, which releases low levels of hydrogen peroxide where the honey makes contact with your wound.[15] The honey makes the wound smell better too.

Manuka honey is made from pollen gathered from the flowers of a medicinal plant called the manuka bush. It is the gold standard in medicinal honey and has been scientifically proven to be antibacterial.[16] However, it's expensive and can be hard to find. You may have just as much luck with raw, unfiltered, local honey as it contains many of the same enzymes. But whatever you do, avoid the highly processed "Grade A" honey you find in most grocery stores. It is more like high fructose corn syrup and is more likely to increase infection.[17] It should never be used to treat wounds.

COOK WITH TURMERIC

Turmeric has been found (not by the FDA, ha ha ha) to reduce inflammation. Many people with HS testify that turmeric helps reduce inflammation and make their boils come to a head faster. In fact, this member of the ginger family is the number one herb recommended on forums and HS support groups.

A lot of people online say that it is the be-all-end-all cure for HS. It's certainly a refreshing alternative to the NSAIDs that increase intestinal permeability.[13]

But turmeric won't stop flare-ups.

Let's face it, my friend: you are probably quite riddled with inflammation from consuming vegetable oils, from not eating enough green leafy vegetables or fish, and from eating grains and legumes and animals that ate grains and legumes. The standard American diet (SAD) is extremely high in omega-6 fatty acids, which are pro-inflammatory. The typical American consumes anywhere between twenty to forty times the optimal 1:1 ratio of omega-3 to omega-6 fatty acids. Such an imbalance is the source of this inflammation. No amount of turmeric will make a dent in that. You simply cannot continue to eat the way you always have and expect a turmeric pill to make it all better.

That said, the compound in turmeric, aka curcumin, has been tested in laboratories to see if it can be of any use in autoimmune diseases. The researchers found some interesting information:

In addition to slowing down the growth of tumors, inflammatory cytokine production, cataract formation, inflammatory bowel disease, and heart disease, heat-solubilized curcumin has been shown to lower cholesterol, suppress diabetes, enhance wound healing, block HIV replication, and modulate multiple sclerosis and Alzheimer's disease.[14]

The scientists involved in the study concluded that curcumin may provide some relief from autoimmune conditions. Here's the catch: *The curcumin they tested was heat-solubilized.* Regular turmeric that you buy at the store or a supplement shop *is not* heat-solubilized. The researchers advised that regular curcumin isn't effective because it is insoluble in water; in other words, it doesn't dissolve. This completely limits its medicinal potential.

There are two things you can do to increase the effectiveness of curcumin. First, cook with it. Curcumin binds to the albumin in eggs quite strongly, so the researchers suggest using turmeric in an omelet. Since egg whites are off the menu in the initial phases of the autoimmune protocol you'll soon be following, you may want to consider the second option: make an infusion (tea) and filter the insoluble turmeric out before you drink it. Don't let it come back to room temperature or you're wasting your time.

And stop wasting your money on turmeric capsules; they won't do a thing except decrease the size of your bank account. However, if you've found that turmeric helps you, there's no reason why you can't continue to take it. In fact, I've got a Turmeric Coffee recipe in the back of this book just for you.

USE SELECT FOLK REMEDIES

Even though traditional medicines seem to have been forgotten by modern medicine, they do have properties that can be useful. Some of the remedies that have lost popularity but are still incredibly useful include *ichthammol salve, iodine tincture,* and *sulfur soap.*

Also known as black drawing salve, ichthammol salve is made from sulfuric shale mixed with a carrier such as paraffin or beeswax. It can be used in the treatment of small wounds to help "draw" out poison, splinters, or toxins. Ichthammol salve is commonly used in folk and natural medicine to help draw out pus and infection from boils. It has also been used with success in the treatment of psoriasis, dermatitis, leg ulcers, and furuncles for over a century.[18] There are no major side effects from Ichthammol salve; however, some people report skin irritation.

BRING ON THE COCONUT OIL

If I could only choose one thing to have in my arsenal against HS, it would be coconut oil. It is amazing on so many levels.

First off, coconut oil is antibacterial, antimicrobial, antiviral, and antifungal. It is also a great moisturizer and conditioner—I even use the stuff on my scalp. You can shave with it, apply it after you've shaved, put it on a new boil, apply it after the boil has burst, and massage it into existing scars. You can eat it to help heal your gut, and thereby heal your skin from the inside.

It's ironic that most of us stay away from products that contain oil, as we mistakenly think that the oil would further clog our pores and create flare-ups. This is not true of coconut oil, at least not for me. I even use it to clean my face before I go to bed at night. I don't use any other products, and I love the way my skin feels.

If you have found an essential oil (for example, tea tree oil) that helps your HS, why not create your very own medicinal lotion using coconut oil? Simply put the coconut oil in a jar, add as much essential oil as you see fit and stir it up. You could add calendula oil, almond oil, goldenseal, or whatever else you would like to the mixture. Store it in the fridge to firm it up if you wish, but refrigeration is not necessary.

> *Healing, Papa would tell me, is not a science, but the intuitive art of wooing nature.*
>
> —W.H. Auden

YES, YOU CAN SHAVE

I'm thankful that I never had HS in my armpits. I've shaved them since I hit puberty and have never had a flare-up there. So, shaving doesn't cause outbreaks.

But it can cause ingrown hairs. Dr. Cordain has identified two different conditions playing a factor in HS, both of which involve the hair follicles.[6] Doing something that intentionally aggravates those hair follicles will not bode well for you while you are having active HS flare-ups. You've probably also noticed that wearing tight clothing, or things that rub against your HS-prone areas like bras can cause boils. Same principle applies.

Tight clothing or rubbing the skin calls attention to that area. Since your immune system is in high alert already, when you shine a light on a specific area, you have more chances of your immune system responding to said area.

That said, areas that have no irritation, rubbing, or attention paid to them can also be prone to HS. Any hair-bearing area on your entire body is a potential target.

Once you've put your HS in remission, you may be able to shave again. You will also notice other changes in your skin. You might not get ingrown hairs from shaving anymore. You'll definitely notice far less inflammation and infection.

If shaving still bothers you, try removing hair by waxing or using a device that pulls hair out by the root. And use a rubbing alcohol wipe or an antiseptic, antimicrobial wipe like Hibiclens directly after shaving or waxing to help prevent ingrown hairs and itching. Apply coconut oil once it's dried. Simply shaving with coconut oil in the first place also helps. It's soothing and an amazing moisturizer.

For the love of God, don't wax or shave an area if you have an active flare-up. The chances of nicking it are astronomical. Instead, take tweezers to the individual hairs right around the boil, so that they don't get caught up in the mess.

EAT BURDOCK ROOT

Burdock root is quite popular in Chinese medicine. It has been used therapeutically in Europe, North America, and Asia for hundreds of years. As a salve, burdock has been used to treat eczema, acne, and psoriasis. As a supplement or food, it has been shown to detoxify the blood and promote circulation.[19] The root also has antioxidant qualities and can help regulate blood sugar.

Burdock seeds have shown the potential to inhibit tumor growth and are also anti-inflammatory. Burdock leaf extract can even stop the growth of microorganisms in your mouth.[20]

Inulin extracted from edible burdock shows prebiotic properties that can help you repopulate your gut flora.[21] Studies show that burdock inulin does not appear to cause bloating, something that is quite common with chicory inulin. As great as this sounds, it is important to be aware that burdock can also cause allergic reactions, including contact dermatitis and inflammatory responses. Tread wisely.

USE HERBAL SCAR CREAMS

If we hear that a particular herb or salve is antibacterial, we're likely to jump on it to try it out for ourselves. If it also helps fade scars, we're sold before we've even tried it. It's so easy to spend hundreds of dollars on lotions and potions, but some of them just don't work. Let's take a look at the ones that do.

Elderberry extract, oregano oil, oregano leaf extract, and golden-seal root have all been proven to have antimicrobial and antibacterial properties, not necessarily killing off the microbes, but definitely inhibiting their growth.[22] Using an herbal cream containing any or all of these ingredients may be very beneficial for a boil that is still in the healing process.

Astragalus, calendula oil, and thyme extract did not live up to expectations in the lab. While they may be good for your skin, they don't actually have any medicinal benefits.

JUST MAKE IT GO AWAY: NUMBING CREAMS

Some people like to use creams from the drugstore that contain pain relieving compounds like benzocaine. I once even asked my dentist for some topical novacaine to help numb a particularly bad boil that wouldn't come to a head. (He said no.) I've used arnica gel and found that I could get about twenty minutes of relief from it, enough to be able to fall asleep. I've used Orajel, which also contains a numbing agent. None of these topical solutions will get rid of a boil (and some of them sting like the dickens), but if you are in a great deal of pain, they may give you some relief. Remember to never use numbing creams on broken skin or after the boil has burst.

DRESS IT UP WITH HYDROCOLLOID DRESSINGS

If you have a particularly painful boil or are trying to avoid infection, you may want to look into hydrocolloid dressings. They're like a really tough, waterproof bandage that sticks to your skin. A great time to use a dressing like this is when the boil is first starting to drain. When the active surface of the dressing comes in contact with fluid or pus, it absorbs it and swells, forming a gel which is held underneath the bandage. The moist conditions under the dressing are intended to promote wound healing, without causing softening or breaking down of the tissue.

Hydrocolloid dressings are sometimes used on the face for acne and for pressure ulcers (bedsores). They don't allow anything in or out, so you can shower with them on or apply a topical medication or salve underneath.

If it doesn't irritate your skin, a padded bandage (like Nexcare brand) can also help. Cleaning the wound and the surrounding skin with rubbing alcohol first and letting it dry before applying the bandage is a fantastic way to make it stick.

Myths & Misconceptions

It's amazing how much crap is out there concerning HS. Misinformation, myths, and old wives tales abound. There are all kinds of crazy theories and medieval-like home remedies (I tried them all), most don't work, some are even downright dangerous. Some wacky treatments work "miracles" for some, but fail miserably for the rest of us. Admit it, you've tried some of them. We all have. We're desperate.

Part of the problem is the Internet. People go online and shout from the rooftops that their HS is cured, after seeing a one-month remission. They credit their remission with some quirky, new thing they tried. They then step out of the room and let the Internet perpetuate itself.

What I have *never* seen is one of these people come back to the HS forums after six months and say, "Hey! My HS is still gone! And all because of that emu oil!"

That's probably because it *isn't* gone anymore. It came back, but they somehow forgot to update their comments.

We are so desperate for an answer, so anxious to find help, that we are willing to try anything. In some cases, these "treatments" cost us hundreds of dollars. In others, they can cause infection or even set back our healing. At best, they're ineffective and a waste of time. There is nothing you can ingest that is going to make your HS *completely better*. To do that, you must heal your gut, period.

Use your common sense when trying out recommendations you find on the Internet—there are *ridiculous* claims out there. I'm not going to deal with most of them. I'm sure you, as an intelligent human being, can see that they're bullshit. My personal favorite claim is that if you rub the night sweat from the back of a toad under a full moon and put it on the boils, they will disappear.

Ummm, OK. I'll get right on that.

Another ludicrous claim I read on the Internet was if you eat twelve chili peppers a day, it'll make your HS go away. This one particularly pisses me off. Not only is this going to be painful, both during ingestion AND elimination, but it could actually make your HS worse. Chili peppers cause and increase intestinal permeability.[23] They are a nightshade. C'mon people, don't fall for this!

There are indeed some crazy myths about HS floating around. Some are popular because they are based in truth. You may have believed some of them yourself, or may still believe them even now.

Over the years, I tried turmeric compresses. I put the messy stuff on the boil and covered it with a Band-Aid. It did nothing except make a terrific mess, especially when the bandage came off during the night and introduced itself to my bed sheets. I can't say it reduced the inflammation in the boil any more than, say, oregano might have.

Nothing else I tried seemed to make any difference either. Using zit cream, antibacterial wash, wart cream (DON'T do this, it's beyond painful), and anything else I could get my hands on had little to no effect, or actually made it worse.

It amazes me the type of things people are willing to put on an open HS lesion in order to "heal" it. Would you smear some dubious salve on your arm if you cut it open with a kitchen knife? I would hope not. However, when I was first learning how to navigate the boils and the healing process I too fell prey to this mindset. I tried anything I heard would work but nothing did. The following pages represent some of the myths some of us have fallen for.

GRAPEFRUIT SEED EXTRACT (GSE)

There have been claims that GSE has antimicrobial, antifungal, and antibacterial effects, but this has never been proven in a laboratory. In fact, multiple scientific studies have found that any antimicrobial activity from GSE is merely from contamination with synthetic antimicrobials and not from the GSE itself.[24] Apart from a pleasant citrus smell, using GSE on your boils won't make a difference, except to your wallet.

COLLOIDAL SILVER

Silver was used to treat wounds before safer measures, such as antibiotics, came onto the scene in the forties. Despite the fact that it has been used for decades, it's effectiveness has never been scientifically proven. In fact, there are studies that show that the use of colloidal silver on external wounds can slow healing.[25] There is also the risk of other side effects, including seizure and death. Most medical authorities and publications advise against the use of colloidal silver.[26]

EMU OIL

There are some companies out there that want to capitalize on your pain and suffering. One recent scandal involved Speer Laboratories, which claimed that its emu oil, Emuaid, would cure HS. The company's founder later released this apology.

> My name is Richard Nicolo and I am the founder of Emuaid and the President of Speer Laboratories. I would like to issue a sincere apology to all of the HS sufferers for the various misrepresentations that were erroneously made on behalf of Emuaid in some advertisements and online posts. It was never our intention to marginalize, mischaracterize or harm anyone in this community. Sadly, HS is a misunderstood condition and we as a company failed to fine-tune our marketing copy to properly address the facts about HS. By no means did we ever intend to imply that HS is communicable or that it could be cured by our product ... we know that it is neither contagious nor curable.[27]

Check out the following Facebook advertisement for Emuaid. Sounds like they were making specific claims to me.

This company wanted to capitalize on the HS market and did so without any hard science to back them up. Thousands of us were fooled. This just goes to show that we're not the only ones who realize how desperate we are.

Emuaid goes for around $50 for a two-ounce jar and also contains colloidal silver and two types of hydrogenated oils.[28] Does it work for HS? Put it this way: the many people I know about who have tried emu oil still have HS. That should be answer enough.

End Hidradentitis Quickly

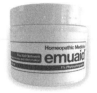

Emuaid© Stops the Bacterial Infection that Causes Hidradenitis and accelerates healing.

WEIRD, FOREIGN HERBS

A lot of us have tried different herbs for our HS, including herbs that claim to reduce inflammation, help with swelling, regulate the immune system, or improve skin and hair. There are thousands of different herbs to choose from, but I have yet to hear of one that works for HS all by itself. Some of them can even be harmful, interact with your hormones, or cause problems of their own.

Cat's Claw

Cat's claw (*Uncaria tomentosa*) grows wild in many countries of Central and South America and has been used for centuries to prevent and treat disease. However, there is not enough scientific evidence to determine whether or not cat's claw is safe in people with conditions that affect the immune system. It can mess up blood pressure during or after surgery and may cause headaches, dizziness, and vomiting. Because it has traditionally been used to help viral infections and it stimulates the immune system, some HS patients put cat's claw on their boils or take it internally. To date, I have not received or read any testimony that shows it works for HS in any way.

Black Seed Oil

Black seed oil (*Nigella sativa Linn*) is also called *black cumin* and *kalonji* and is used for medicinal purposes all over the world. Black seed oil is even mentioned in the Bible and the Quran as a cure-all. It is supposed to have anti-inflammatory, fever reducing, pain relieving, and germ fighting properties; it's even supposed to lower cholesterol. HS sufferers may take it for any of these reasons, but especially because it is supposed to balance the immune system.

Unfortunately I was not able to find a single medical study that could remotely prove any of these things. In fact, the one study I did find said that "cytokine production of ... mice that were given *Nigella sativa Linn* for thirty days was not significantly different than those who took saline solution instead."[29]

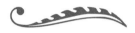

The Bottom Line

Forget about all the dubious claims out there and be smart about where your money goes. Spending cash on quality food will go much further to helping your HS than buying strange potions or pills.

CHAPTER SEVEN
Dealing With Stress

> *To keep the body in good health is a duty... otherwise we shall not be able to keep our mind strong and clear.*
> —Buddha

Since the 1950s, the word *stress*—and the ever-complicated campaign to rid ourselves of it—has become enmeshed in our culture. Our bodies generally don't like stress. It makes us overeat, tired, irritable, and frustrated. The fallout from a poor diet, lack of exercise, and the frenetic lives we lead can result in health problems like weight gain, high blood pressure, loss of libido, and even death.

Every time we're stuck in traffic or get cut off, our blood pressure raises and our stress hormones are released. Every time we get on a treadmill, we send our body a signal that we're in danger and must outrun a predator (I mean, come on, why else would we run? For enjoyment?! Ha.). If we don't sleep enough, fuel our body properly, or don't take the time to play, rest, and relax, our body reads that as stress. Add financial burdens or family problems to the mix and you have the worst kind stress of all: the chronic and long-term kind.

Many people with HS see a correlation between their flare-ups and how stressed out they are. True, stress does play a factor in autoimmune disease flare-ups,[1] but it is *only part of the chain* (albeit, an *important* part of the chain). Stress causes a series of reactions within the body that can result in a flare-up, if all the other stars align—that is, your genes, gut, and environment are all working against you at the same time.

Reducing the amount of negative stress in your life is imperative if you want to achieve remission. Unfortunately it is way beyond the scope of this book to fix all the stressors in your life. I'm not going to recommend any touchy-feely office workshop crap about sharing your feelings or squeezing a ball to reduce stress, either. Those are recommendations from people who don't get it. Besides, as we'll soon find out, a lot of your stress is actually caused by your leaky gut. Squeezing a ball is not going to fix a leaky gut.

My guess is that your HS is probably one of the biggest stressors in your life. It certainly was in mine. Let's find out what part stress plays— and doesn't play— in autoimmune conditions.

The Mind-Gut Connection

That stress can bring on a flare-up probably comes as no surprise. Many of us are all too aware that our state of mind can have a huge influence over our bodies. Think about the last time you salivated over food before it had even touched your lips. Just the sight of it, even the mere thought, can bring on such a reaction. This is a sign that your mind anticipates receiving that food and in preparation to do so, instructs your body to release digestive enzymes. Conversely, if you're nervous, you may find that your stomach gets upset or you may even lose your appetite.

What you may not realize is the mind-gut connection works both ways: the gut can also have a direct effect on the brain. For example, when your gut is leaky and inflamed, those wonderful chemical messengers, the inflammatory cytokines we've learned so much about, travel from the gut by way of the bloodstream and activate the brain's resident immune cells. There, the cytokines initiate low-level inflammation. An inflamed brain can manifest as stress, depression, or anxiety.[2]

Such strong negative emotions ultimately end up decreasing the blood flow to the intestine and suppressing the intestinal immune system.[3] This causes inflammation in the gut, problems with digestion, bacterial overgrowth, and eventually, a leaky gut. It's a vicious circle.

When we experience stress, the sympathetic nervous system takes over. This is also known as "fight or flight." If you continue to activate your fight-or-flight response, you will continue to experience inflammation.[4] This will delay your healing—or possibly even prevent it.

To top it off, when your intestines are damaged and inflamed, your body produces less of the neurotransmitter serotonin—which is involved in mood control, depression, and aggression. Though produced in the brain, the greatest concentration of serotonin takes place in the gut, and when levels drop, you end up feeling even more down and depressed—a literal circle of strife.

So, if stress is causing your leaky gut, and the leaky gut is causing your depression, then adding a heaping handful of your trigger foods into the mix will wreak havoc. As you begin to heal your gut, you may start to feel better mentally—more focused, energetic, and happy. This is your clue that things are working.

The New Prozac

I know we covered probiotics earlier in our discussion on dysbiosis, but I just can't get enough of them. And neither should you. Probiotics are the most powerful weapon in your arsenal against HS, other autoimmune conditions, and even mental problems like depression, anxiety, and ADHD. Many people suffering from HS also suffer from depression. When we look at the primary cause of HS—a leaky gut—it's easy to see why.

Growing research indicates that the bacteria living in your gut play major roles in the development of brain, behavioral, and emotional

STRESSED & HS-FREE

At the time of this writing, I'm sitting here with $26 in the bank, thousands in debt, with a husband who just deployed for two months leaving me with three-year-old twin boys who are in that horrible independent-tantrum stage and who won't even let me go to the bathroom by myself. I am not sleeping enough, I am hung-over from going out drinking for my birthday, and I am anxious about not being able to buy toilet paper next week. I would say in the grand scheme of things, I'm pretty stressed out.

But I am still HS free. If stress alone caused HS, I would be riddled with boils. Like hormones and sugar, stress is involved in the equation but it is not the sole cause of your HS.

Now, if I were to do some good ol' comfort eating (something with mashed potatoes or spaghetti and bread, say) right before my period plus throw in the stress, we would have a different outcome altogether.

problems.[5] It turns out taking probiotics doesn't just make for short bathroom visits—it also helps control anxiety and depression because probiotics affect our neurotransmitters.[6] Antidepressants work by increasing the amount of serotonin in the brain, but do not address serotonin deficiencies in the gut, which is why they rarely work.[7] Simply taking probiotic supplements for four short weeks can improve your mood, attention, response to sensation, and emotional behavior.[8]

I simply cannot overemphasize the value of taking probiotics to improve gut flora, which also helps us out by affecting energy balance, glucose metabolism, and low-grade inflammation.[9]

Now, we've talked a lot about *gut* flora, but you should also be aware that bacteria help protect *all* of the mucous membranes in your body. That includes your eyes, nose, mouth, windpipe, lungs, urethra, and urinary bladder as well as your stomach and intestines. Oh, and did I forget to mention your skin? Your body is teeming with bacteria—some good, some bad. The modern impulse is to sterilize ourselves and our environment—to kill off absolutely everything—but research is starting to emerge that perhaps that isn't such a great idea.

Researchers at the National Institutes of Health Human Microbiome Project (HMP) and others at companies like uBiome are furiously working to map the microbial communities found at several different places on the human body, including nasal passages, oral cavities, the skin, the urogenital tract as well as the gastrointestinal tract, to see what role these microbes play in human health and disease. Scientists have already discovered that many chronic conditions and symptoms are caused by an overgrowth of bad bacteria—and a lack of beneficial bacteria to keep them in check.[10]

Many of us suffer from HS flare-ups inside our noses. (You may have thought that you had ingrown hairs, but let me school you, honey: *anywhere* you have a hair follicle, you can have an HS flare.) You may also be suffering from chronic sinusitis or allergies. Along with body-wide inflammation and autoimmune responses, if you're having problems with your nose, you probably have *sinus dysbiosis*. (As a side note, if you suffer from sinusitis, repopulating your sinus flora by adding a little bit of probiotic to your neti pot is tremendously effective. My chronic sinusitis and seasonal allergy symptoms disappeared after only three applications.)

Maintaining the integrity of microbial communities in *all* the mucous membranes of your body is just as important as making sure your gut flora is rockin' and rollin'. The microbes on your skin may play a part in how bad your HS flare-ups end up being, resulting in infection and that really bad smell some of us have come to associate with HS. After all, opportunistic bacteria cause body odor. Just something to think about the next time you're reaching for antibiotic cream to slather all over your butt.[11]

Historically, probiotics were a regular part of our daily diet. Before we had refrigerators, we fermented foods to preserve them. Most traditional cultures served some sort of fermented food every day—whether it was sauerkraut, kimchi, or kefir depended on where you lived. Fermented foods are one of those borderline foods for us—they can be healing to the gut, but potentially hazardous if yeast is one of our triggers. We'll explore fermented foods in greater depth in chapters eight and nine.

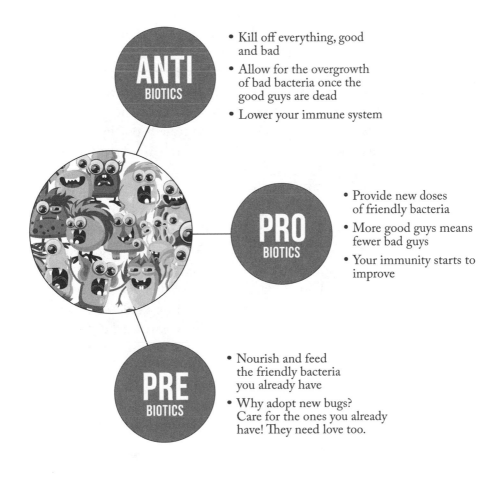

ANTI BIOTICS
- Kill off everything, good and bad
- Allow for the overgrowth of bad bacteria once the good guys are dead
- Lower your immune system

PRO BIOTICS
- Provide new doses of friendly bacteria
- More good guys means fewer bad guys
- Your immunity starts to improve

PRE BIOTICS
- Nourish and feed the friendly bacteria you already have
- Why adopt new bugs? Care for the ones you already have! They need love too.

Stress Management

Changing your diet and introducing probiotics will instantly make you feel less stressed out. You'll find that your body and mind can handle just about anything you throw at it. Here are a couple other things that you can do to help yourself manage stress better.

SLEEP

Sleep is critically important but it's something that we tend to abuse. We stay up long after the sun has gone down and wake up to hideous alarms that jolt us out of dreamland (our bodies see this signal as an alarm all right—one that means we'd better run for our lives or be eaten or maimed). Our bodies need rest in order to reset and repair. If you are not sleeping enough, you will have elevated cortisol levels, which is the number one indicator of stress. Excess cortisol can make you gain weight, especially around the middle where it's most dangerous. Lack of sleep also lowers your immune system.

Ideally, you want to go to bed when it gets dark and get up with the sun. If you can't do that, try to go to bed as early as you can, in a completely darkened room. Avoid exposure to electronics and bright lights for an hour or two before bed. Light exposure tells our hypothalamus that it's daytime, and melatonin production (an important hormone that makes us sleepy) is affected.

If you have trouble falling asleep or your circadian rhythm is completely messed up, you can take melatonin tablets an hour or so before you want to be asleep. Make sure you avoid bright light and electronics after you've taken the melatonin, though. We've all experienced overriding our body's natural melatonin at some point—I call it "getting my second wind" when I go out late at night. Any disruption in routine or lighting can also override the melatonin—if we couldn't get up in a hurry or stay awake in an emergency, we'd likely have died out eons ago. You'll be wasting your time if you take the supplement and don't crawl into bed soon thereafter.

Try to get (on average) eight to nine hours of sleep a night. That's right, eight to nine. In the winter, you may find you want to sleep more. Do it. Try to get up without an alarm on days when it's not critical for you to be up at the crack of dawn.

Once you start sleeping more, you will feel better during the day, have way more energy, and handle any stress that comes your way. Add the next element, exercise, and you will feel like a kid again.

Sleep affects every aspect of your life. If you don't sleep properly, it will cascade into other areas of your life without you even noticing. Take it seriously or it will take you out.

EXERCISE

This is a tricky one. At least *some* level of exercise is absolutely critical. Too little and it's just not effective. If you overdo it, your body thinks you're stressed out.

As we've just learned, stress can cause leaky gut. Exercise itself directly causes leaky gut too. For years, professional athletes who perform high-intensity exercises have been experiencing something called *exercise-induced intestinal barrier dysfunction.*[12]

Your body also sees the wrong *type* of exercise as stress. We thrive when our genes are given what they've evolved to expect: the right food, proper sleep, and primal movements like thrusting, lifting, climbing, and chopping. There's a reason everyone in that Globo-gym down the street from you looks the same year after cardio-filled year. They are not moving in a way their bodies understand as beneficial. According to their brains (and their second brains, i.e., their guts) these people are being chased by a saber-toothed tiger for sixty minutes, four times a week.

On the flipside, exercise gives us energy and releases chemicals in our brains that make us happy—it's good for us in a lot of ways. It makes us more sensitive to insulin, meaning that the skin cells around our hair follicles won't be as prone to growing out of control. When you become more insulin sensitive, your body will naturally produce more *sex hormone binding globulin* (SHBG), the hormone we discussed back in chapter five that binds to free testosterone. Gentle exercise also reduces the amount of cortisol our bodies produce, thereby lowering the amount of progesterone in the blood.

> I've reduced a lot of the stress in my life. I've gotten rid of a lot of things. The light was turned on, and a lot of the cockroaches started spinning. I swept them out the door. And sometimes you just have to throw things out, because they carry a certain energy.
>
> —Wesley Snipes

It helps to reduce inflammation, lower the amount of pro-inflammatory cytokines we produce, and just generally make life worth living.

So, if too much exercise is bad, and the wrong type is bad, but we still have to do *some*, how on earth do we find a happy medium and do what's right? The answer: the exact same way we find out what we should eat. We look to our ancestors.

Primal Movements

Imagine a time before there were cars to transport us, machines to do the heavy lifting, and factories producing our food. What did we *do* all day? We didn't sit on our bums, that's for sure.

Early modern man moved a lot. They built shelters, gathered food, hunted, played, carried heavy things, and did whatever else was necessary. They had short bursts of high-intensity movement—for example, running away from a tiger or chopping down a tree—and when there was nothing else to do, they basically just took it easy.

It's in our nature to rest. That's part of what makes it so hard to stick with modern exercise routines like step aerobics. There's no real purpose to them, and you've got nothing to show for your hard work when you're done. Why on earth would your primal brain want to continue a useless, fruitless activity for more than, say, two weeks?

In order to make exercise sustainable, you need to make it enjoyable—and useful. If taking down a moose or a tree is not exactly your idea of enjoyment, it's easy enough to *trick* your body into thinking it's doing something useful. This is where primal movement patterns come into play.

Walking, sprinting, pushing, pulling, throwing, thrusting, squatting, lunging, climbing, and jumping are all great examples. These are full-body movements that have real world applications. Such activities are not considered negative stressors because your genes recognize them as normal. Moving the way your body expects you to move seems to unlock some hidden door deep within our genetic code. Not only does this type of exercise alleviate common injuries and pain associated with moving incorrectly, this gene expression seems to accelerate weight loss.

Where you exercise is also really important. Our ancestors didn't move around all day in windowless boxes, staring at images of themselves while listening to heavy metal and ignoring everyone around them. Getting outside in the sunshine will make the difference between a workout that helps you unwind and one that leaves you feeling drained.

Lifting weights using functional movements and other strength training exercises are generally good ways to improve stress. So are short sprints. Exercising or playing games with other people is also a great way to improve your mood.

Gentle walking most days and higher intensity primal movements about two to three times a week should be about all you need if your goal is stress reduction and general health. If you're looking to compete in the CrossFit games, obviously your schedule will look a little different.

Listening to the signals your body sends you is also very important. If you don't feel like working out, don't. When you feel like moving, *move*. If you can get your exercise in by doing something useful, it'll be easier to stick with and you'll feel better afterwards. I personally think walking to the store and carrying groceries home is a very useful workout indeed.

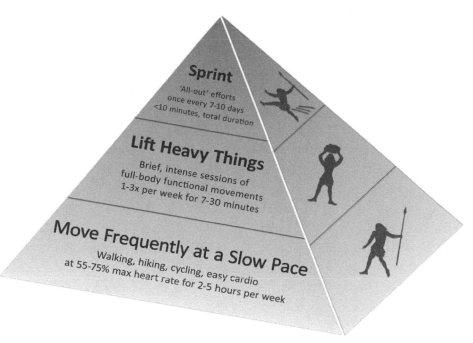

Image provided courtesy of Primal Blueprint, Inc.

SEX

Most of us don't do this enough, especially if we're married. Sex is one of the best ways to bond with your partner and foster feelings of security and love, and can help you through times of stress and hardship.

Orgasm releases a wave of chemicals in our brains that is similar to exercise, but more potent. The surge of oxytocin, the "cuddle hormone" that occurs with orgasm, has been shown to lower blood pressure, help you sleep better, and reduce stress.[13]

If you don't have a partner, don't let that stop you. Self-love is almost as effective, and you'll want to cuddle with yourself afterwards. That's always nice.

As far as I know, there are no links between sex and leaky gut. Unless you smoke afterwards.

NEW AGE-Y STUFF

Some people find a huge reduction in their stress levels with meditation and yoga. While I love yoga and often feel like I've had a good nap when I've finished practicing, meditation just isn't for me.

All you're really trying to achieve when you meditate or practice yoga is to bring yourself into the present moment and to tune everything else out. It's easy to do this other ways.

If you find that you're not able to meditate while sitting in a quiet, comfortable place, don't worry about it. I "meditate" whenever I find myself in the woods and sometimes even when I'm eating. There are no rules that say you have to close your eyes and hum. In fact, there are no rules at all. Do whatever works for you. Taking in the beauty of nature and fresh air is usually enough for me. Combining this with the rhythmic pace of walking and deep breathing works wonders. If I'm in a stressful situation, taking a few long, slow breaths is often enough. Years ago, I smoked to relieve stress. But now I realize it was probably the deep breathing that helped me relax, not the tobacco.

The same is true of yoga. Yoga forces you to breath deeply, to pay attention to your body, and to be in the present moment (or you'll fall over on your butt). Gentle stretching with attention to breathing can bring many of the same benefits as being twisted into a pretzel can.

GET RID OF TOXIC PEOPLE

Maybe there are people in your life who make you feel bad about yourself, your situation, the movie you just watched, the clothes you picked out, or the car you drive. It doesn't seem to matter what you do or what's going on in the world, these are the sort of people who leave you feeling bad about yourself.

Sometimes they don't consciously mean to. Sometimes they do. Whatever their motivations, the end result is the same. Like vampires, they suck the emotional energy right out of you. Their behavior can manifest as sabotage, condescension, irritation, or abuse. Regardless, the lasting impact can be depressing and stressful.

Tossing toxic people like this to the curb can be an immense stress reliever. No longer having to worry about what they'll think, or feeling dread over the thought of meeting up with them, will go a long way toward making you feel better. If you truly care for a toxic person (or they're family and you can't get rid of them), talking to them about how they make you feel can sometimes help. If it doesn't, try to limit the amount of time and energy you spend on them.

TAKE TIME FOR YOURSELF

However appealing the idea, making time for ourselves is often hard. If you find you give all your energy to others in your life, and rarely have time to breathe, try scheduling a relaxing activity for yourself. Treat it as you would any other appointment and you'll be sure to go.

Other things that have been found to reduce stress include pets, playing games, and reconnecting with nature. A hike through the forest or a walk on the beach will do wonders for both your state of mind and your cortisol levels. Bring along your dog and a ball, and you've got all three elements covered.

MAKE DECISIONS FOR YOURSELF

As you embark upon your journey, you'll find that you alone hold the key to healing yourself from HS. Decisions that you make each and every day have consequences that may take months to heal from later. I'm not just talking about food; I'm referring to all aspects of your life. Online forums, friends, and family are great sources of support, but at the end of the day, you will have to rely on yourself and your intuition most of the time.

When we flare up for no apparent reason, it is easy to fall into victim mode and isolate ourselves from friends, family, and social situations. Instead of becoming despondent over what seems like a terrible situation over which you have no control, use flare-ups as motivation. Look closely at the choices you have made recently. Scour your food journal to see if there's something you can change. Be honest with yourself about your stress level and how you're handling it. You have complete power in this situation—in fact, you are the only one that does. Being a victim helps no one. Neither does giving your power away.

Rely on your gut feeling about things. There are a few questions you can ask yourself, if you're not sure what to do, take, eat, or be associated with:

Is this going to contribute to or delay my healing?

Does this cause or reduce inflammation?

Will I upset someone if I don't do this? Is placating them more important than causing harm to myself?

Have I read any medical studies on this? Or am I relying on second hand information from the media, doctors, or other sources I can't be sure of?

If I do this, will I feel better or worse later?

Am I actually in a position to make a rational decision about this now, or should I sleep on it?

Taking the time to ask yourself these simple questions can help you avoid impulsive decisions, giving into temporary cravings or wasting time and money.

GET RID OF TOXINS

Toxins from our diet and the environment put added stress on our bodies and our minds. Whether they come in the form of phytohormones, FDA-approved food-grade artificial chemicals or fumes from cleaning supplies, anything toxic in our life is something that our body needs to process and get rid of.

Certain food additives that are common in the United States have been banned in other countries because they have been deemed unsafe. Examples of this include the artificial colors Blue 1, Blue 2, Yellow 6, and Red 40. When I lived in Germany, I could not find a single product that contained high fructose corn syrup, either. I was told the government had ruled it "unfit for human consumption." They didn't consider it safe enough to enter the food supply.

Added stress to our liver and kidney from artificial foods, chemicals, and toxins ultimately results in added stress to us. Take a good look around at your environment and see what you can get rid of today.

Toxins and chemicals aren't the only things we need to be concerned about when it comes to our diet. Other foods that are seemingly harmless can also be causing stress to our body and mind.

Let's move on now and find out the best way to discover what your food triggers are in the next section, *The HS Autoimmune Protocol.*

THE HS-DIET CONNECTION

As HS sufferers started writing in with success stories, it became clear that we share some common triggers, and that some of us have triggers that are uniquely ours. These can be particularly hard to pinpoint, requiring a little more detective work. Nonetheless, there's no denying the connection between our diet and the state of our skin, as the following testimonies will attest.

Laura: I also had breakouts on [my] buttocks and under [my] breasts. Switched to eating Primal 90 percent and [the breakouts] cleared up. Ditched raw tomatoes also.

Missy: It has become more clear to me over the years that the triggers were there, but hard to identify. This year I was diagnosed with silent reflux, and now I am seeing a relationship between trigger foods in both conditions. Tomatoes, for sure....

Kate: Mine got better dramatically when I was on the hCG [41] diet without carbs, although I have since fallen off that wagon. Am working my way up to full Paleo. Nightshades are definitely out next.

Michelle: The autoimmune paleo lifestyle has all but cured me of [my HS]; very rarely I'll get a flat red circle a couple times a year. About ten years ago I was on a very non-paleo low carb diet and found that Splenda caused terrible HS breakouts. Next worse were tomatoes.

Kori: I too have suffered (continue to suffer) from HS since puberty. Since going Primal, I have noticed a severe reduction in outbreaks but not a total remission. It is true that diet has been key. I have bad flare-ups once or twice a year now as opposed to once a month.

Barb: For the last twenty years I have tried to define what was making me break out like the measles, and lasting for weeks on end. Leaving scars [on the] backs of my thighs, head, arms … a real mess. Always thought it was nuts, but since pulling out the nightshades, the spots are healing and [I'm] not getting new ones.

Katie: I truly believe that an autoimmune/Primal/paleo diet does greatly improve issues. I really appreciate the mindset of the Primal/paleo community over the disease-based diet groups. The diseased-based diet folks often seem to take a victim role of 'I am damaged and can eat only these foods.' Whereas the Primal/Paleo folks seem to take the approach of 'I am going to have a vibrant life, and these foods are damaging so I don't want to eat them.' A very powerful difference.

PART TWO:

THE HS AUTOIMMUNE PROTOCOL

CHAPTER EIGHT

Phase I: The Elimination Diet

By now, you should have a pretty good understanding which foods can cause leaky gut, how autoimmunity factors into the equation, and the roles that stress and hormones play. We're now going to move on to what you can eat. Finally.

The foods you will be eating are based on the diets of our Paleolithic ancestors. You may have heard it referred to as Primal or paleo or ancestral, but essentially you'll be eating the foods that your body evolved to thrive upon. One side effect of eating this way is weight loss. Another is vibrant health and energy. Yet another is clear skin and silky hair. Once you start to see some of these and other benefits, it will be a lot easier to stick to it.

But first, we'll start off with an elimination test, designed to jump-start the healing process of your gut and ultimately your skin. For thirty to sixty days, you will be cutting a whole lot of foods out of your life. These include all the foods that lead to leaky gut syndrome (reviewed in chapter four) and all the foods that commonly trigger flare-ups. The foods you are left with will form the foundation of your personalized ancestral diet, which you will begin to build as you reintroduce certain foods back into your diet.

In the next chapter, we will discuss the reintroduction phase in greater depth. It is designed to zero in and find the trigger foods that give you boils. In this phase, you will monitor your body's reaction to certain foods as you gradually introduce them one at a time back into your diet. This is how you will find your personal triggers. In this phase, you will learn which foods you can permanently welcome back, which you can tolerate in small amounts, and which you must always avoid. From these experiments, you will build your personalized "diet." You'll have no idea what to call this new diet, and it won't matter. It will be what you make it. It will become as individual as you are.

I suggest thirty to sixty days in the elimination phase, but only you will know when you're ready to move on and begin the next phase. There are many individual factors involved, including how bad your HS is, what other autoimmune conditions you're suffering from, and how long you've been suffering. Since your body needs to do a great deal of healing and reduce inflammation, you may want to wait until it's been at least four weeks without a flare-up before you move on. If you are a woman, it may be a good idea to wait until after you've completed your monthly cycle to see if there are significant changes. Do not attempt to reintroduce foods if you are still flaring up.

During the elimination phase, you may get bored. You may eat the same things over and over again. You won't be able to eat anything packaged or pre-made for a while—convenience foods are out. So is the birthday cake your coworkers ordered especially for you. Even one little cheat can set you back to day one. Sounds hard, doesn't it? It can be if you aren't truly dedicated.

But I can tell you this: while you spend way more time than normal in the kitchen lovingly preparing food for yourself, you will have a lot of time to think about how freakin' awesome you feel. And you may discover something new about yourself too. You may find yourself becoming more adventurous in the kitchen, scouring the Internet in search of what you can do with some random, new vegetable, say a kohlrabi, or how to use fresh herbs to make your burger or chicken more exciting. You may save some money by not eating out anymore and you may even meet new friends. Remember, there is a whole community of people just like you who are working through the same issues that you are. Even if you are unable to get the support you need at home, you can find it elsewhere. Consider this your personal invitation to join the PrimalGirl.com forum. I'm hoping that you will be among the growing online community of HS sufferers who support each other and share their success stories, recipes, and advice.

To be sure, navigating an autoimmune diet can be tricky. It will seem at first that all your favorites are off the menu. With time, you'll come up with some replacements. Things will also get easier once the initial cravings have subsided (about three weeks). Also, once you've ruled out certain foods as triggers, you'll be able to eat them again. It'll only take a couple months of elimination before this happens.

C'mon, don't you think clear, smooth skin and a pain-free life is worth a couple of months of not being able to eat ketchup? I certainly do.

Although the elimination phase of this process may seem overwhelming at first, it is important to remember that it won't last forever. A couple months out of your life really aren't that long, especially if you consider how long you've been dealing with HS. Besides, you'll be able to add a lot of things back in after a while, being absolutely sure that they aren't affecting you negatively. Knowing exactly how your body responds to different foods can be incredibly empowering.

I suggest that you refrain from reintroducing foods during this period, no matter how much you may crave them. Although you may suspect that some of these foods are not direct triggers for your HS, they will affect how quickly your gut heals and interfere with the food experiments that you will conduct in the reintroduction phase.

Besides, until you go through a meticulous elimination diet and evaluate their effects on you when they are reintroduced, you really cannot know for sure what foods are safe for you. It seems logical to think that there's no way that something you have been eating for longer than you've had HS could be the culprit, right? Wrong!

Don't discount a food you've eaten since birth as the cause of your HS. While I was growing up, my family ate a lot of potatoes. I never considered potatoes to be a problem because they were a staple in our household, nothing new or exotic. They were a part of my life long before the HS arrived.

But it turns out that they were the problem. At least part of it.

The entire nightshade family poses a problem for me, along with wheat and yeast, all of which I had been eating since my mom introduced solids foods to me.

I've only in recent years discovered that potatoes give me flare-ups on my buttocks, tomatoes give me flare-ups on my face, and peppers give me inflamed ingrown hairs (especially in my nose). Tobacco creates systemic inflammation and just seems to make everything worse. I don't know what eggplant does, because I cannot stomach the thought of ever eating it again. Point is, I would not have known any of this without first eliminating nightshades from my diet and later experimenting with their return.

Furthermore, we can (and do) develop allergies and intolerances as we grow older.[1] People seem to think that if they weren't allergic to a certain food as a child, they never will be. That's just not true. I watched my husband, who never had an allergy a day in his life, all of a sudden develop seasonal allergies. We were living in the same place where he grew up, so it didn't make any sense. Once he removed wheat and legumes from his diet and allowed his gut to heal, his allergies went away. As an added benefit to his diet change, his IBS went away too.

Fact is, your body changes over the years, depending on your eating and lifestyle habits. I myself developed season allergies at the age of twenty-four. Over time, your body's response to proteins and allergens can change.[2] I like to think of it as an evolution: your body sends you signals, you ignore them (or put on cream or take pills), then there are more warning signs—maybe fatigue or joint pains—and you ignore those too. Additional symptoms arise and the madness continues, until finally your body gets your attention with a symptom so severe you are forced to take notice. That's usually the time all hell breaks loose. Though this picture is not very scientific or doctor-y, it is probably pretty accurate.

If I look back at my early childhood, I had many signs and symptoms of insulin-resistance that went ignored. When I was eight years old, I suddenly became ten pounds overweight and remained at least ten pounds overweight well into my adult years. When I was nine, I became near-sighted and needed glasses.[3] At puberty, I had horrific mood swings and cystic acne. Once I began menstruating, my periods were never regular and were terribly painful. The HS started soon after I started menstruating. The whole time, I was itchy or had mysterious bug bites that no one else seemed to get. It would be years later—overweight and in stage II HS—before I began to turn it all around with diet.

Now it's your turn. Your first step on the road to better health begins with eliminating the antinutrient foods we discussed back in chapter four, *Follow Your Gut*. In addition to those foods, we'll be eliminating a few other items commonly known to trigger HS.

When you first change your diet, I recommend eating simple meals of protein and vegetables for a few weeks. Avoid baking if you can, as most recipes call for eggs. Once you've decided to start adding things back in, you can try some paleo baking and reintroduce nuts and eggs to see how you react.

If your gut is particularly sensitive, I suggest removing the peels from fruits and vegetables. They are the plant's natural barrier against insects and contain varying amounts of antinutrients that can make your tummy rumbly. This especially applies to root vegetables.

When choosing foods, please go for quality over quantity whenever possible. Choosing organic fruits and vegetables and naturally raised meats will equate to a healthier you.

The list of foods on the next page may appear limited, but rest assured that as you explore the world of ancestral eating, you will discover a whole host of exciting new foods and recipes. There are literally hundreds of different types of meat, vegetables, leafy greens, tubers, and low-glycemic fruits at your disposal. And don't forget fresh herbs and seasonings.

You really are limited only by your imagination. Ancestral eating has taken off in recent years, and as a result, there has been an explosion of cookbooks and websites dedicated to the Primal/paleo lifestyle. Be sure to explore these options. The recipes are all gluten-free and many are free of yeast, nightshades, and pseudo grains. And don't forget to check out the tips and recipes in chapter ten.

Now, let's take a closer look at the menu for the next month or so. If you are unsure of a certain food item that is not on this list, go online and research it on one of the many Primal/paleo sites such as Paleo-Hacks.com. If you can't find an answer, err on the side of caution.

Foods You Can Eat Freely

PROTEIN
Any type of meat, including beef, pork, fish, wild game, and fowl

FAT
Tallow, lard, coconut oil, ghee, avocado oil, olive oil,
palm shortening, and avocados

CARBOHYDRATE
Vegetables, leafy greens, most root vegetables and tubers,
and some fruits

MISCELLANEOUS
Coconut, stevia, herbs, and non-seed based spices that aren't derived
from nightshades. Coffee and tea are fine, but proceed with caution:
they can be contaminated with wild yeast or mycotoxins.

Items to Eliminate First

Alcohol
Chemicals
Dairy
Eggs
Grains, pseudo grains, legumes
Nightshades, including tobacco, certain spices
Polyunsaturated vegetable oils
Prepackaged and processed convenience foods
Seeds
Sugar, fruit juice, dried fruit, jams, syrups
Splenda and other artificial sweeteners
Yeast in all forms, including mushrooms, truffles, fermented foods

Items to Eliminate Last

Coffee, chocolate, nuts, salt

Foods You Can Eat Freely

PROTEIN

Meat

Choose the best options that you can afford. Although grass-fed beef is more expensive than conventionally raised beef, it's a great source of omega-3 fatty acids. Conventionally raised animals are fed corn, wheat, and soy, and injected with hormones and antibiotics—meaning that you're eating that garbage too. Also, try expanding your horizons. How long has it been since you've eaten duck or lamb? Ever tried goat, ostrich, caribou, or wild game? You may have to get creative in finding some of the more exotic proteins out there. If you hunt, or have a friend who hunts, getting these meats will be easier for you. If you don't, check out the resources chapter at the back of the book for ideas on where to find them.

Bacon

It's a bit of a joke how much paleo people like their bacon. We even have t-shirts that say, "Bacon is rad. Gluten is bad." (That's right, we have t-shirts.) Look for organic, free-range, cruelty-free bacon that has no added nitrates, chemicals, or sugar in it. Forget about soy bacon and other frankenfoods. Even foods like turkey bacon are processed, loaded with chemicals, and full of sugar. We're not worried about fat content anymore and we're trying to eat real food, so stick to the natural stuff. Don't throw the fat away, either! Sauté your vegetables in it for an amazing burst of flavor. I also fry eggs in it and have even added it to my coffee. The recipe for Bacon Lattes is included in chapter ten.

Bone broth

The nutrients and minerals in homemade broth are not only super good for you, they can help heal the lining of your gut. Store-bought broth doesn't contain these nutrients and, comparatively speaking, is ridiculously expensive. I make up gallons of broth at a time and freeze it in one-cup amounts so it's ready whenever I need it. Be sure to check out the recipe for homemade bone broth on page 204.

FATS
Tallow and lard
It bears repeating: do not fear saturated fats! They help fight infection, aid digestion, and contain loads of omega-3 fats. But let's be clear: I'm not talking about the hydrogenated crap you see on the shelves of the grocery store—I'm talking about real, organic tallow (beef fat) and lard (pig fat) that you've rendered down yourself, from grass-fed, free-range animals. The same thing your grandparents used to cook with. Good ole fashioned fat. I use both tallow and lard to deep fry things like zucchini, taro root, and sweet potatoes. Yum!

Duck fat
If you are lucky enough to spot rendered duck fat at a grocery store, I suggest you buy every single carton in stock immediately. Once you've tried it, you will understand. Vegetables—especially root vegetables—sautéed in duck fat are in a class of their own.

Ghee
Organic ghee (clarified butter) is also a great alternative to regular butter as it doesn't contain the milk proteins that most people react to when they react to butter. Grass-fed organic ghee is available online (please see resources at the end of the book) and in some stores. Ghee can be used in place of butter in most recipes or when you're sautéing things. Use the same amount as you would butter.

Coconut oil
Coconut oil is about 90 percent saturated fat, and has been used for generations in countries like the Philippines, India, and Thailand with no adverse side effects. In fact, research now shows that the benefits of coconut oil far outweigh any mythical problems. With its regained popularity, you can now find it in virtually every grocery store as well as online. It contains medium-chain triglycerides (MCTs), which are easy to absorb and digest. MCTs move easily through the blood and into the liver where they're quickly converted into energy. They also suppress inflammation and repair tissue as well as help neutralize the bad guys like *H-pylori, candida albicans*, and *giardia*.[4] All good things for your leaky gut. The lauric acid in coconut oil turns into monolaurin

once it reaches your intestines and is a very powerful antimicrobial agent. Coconut oil can actually prevent heart disease, is used to reduce stress, is helpful for skin problems, and can increase immunity.

I use coconut oil to cook with, to bake with, and I eat it straight out of the jar. It's great instead of butter, in coffee, and even as a preconditioning treatment for hair. It's a fantastic moisturizer, too. If you aren't using coconut oil yet, get on it. You won't regret it.

CARBOHYDRATES
Vegetables
The standard American diet contains about six different vegetables: potatoes, carrots, peas, lima beans, corn, and ketchup. Problem is, four of these items aren't vegetables at all, and they are all are very high on the glycemic index. Worse of all, five of these six foods can cause leaky gut, digestive upset, and autoimmune conditions. Can you guess which ones? If not, refer back to chapter four, *Follow Your Gut.*

Be adventurous when you're at the farmers market or grocery store and try new vegetables. If you're not sure how to cook them, look up recipes online and experiment. My family regularly eats spinach, broccoli, carrots, sweet potatoes, brussels sprouts, celery, onions, cucumber, winter squash, summer squash, cauliflower, artichoke, kale, chard, lettuce, taro root, celery root, kohlrabi, and parsnips. Get creative; there is more to life than potatoes and peas.

Sweet potatoes and other tubers
Sweet potatoes and yams are not in the nightshade family and are safe replacements for white potatoes. Like potatoes, they are root vegetables and are full of all the same starchy goodness. There are sweet potato and root vegetable chips on the market or you can make your own if you get a deep fryer. Use organic lard (pork fat), tallow (beef fat), coconut or palm oil to fry them in and you'll reap the health benefits as well as impart an amazing flavor. Keep any packaged chips to a minimum; even if they don't have nightshades in them, they're still fried in vegetable oil, which can increase inflammation in your body.

I've experimented with different root vegetables and have found they're all delicious baked, fried, or boiled. Root vegetables that have a similar color and taste to potatoes are taro and yuca root. Don't be frightened by these things if you've never worked with them. They're very easy to make. You'll find some tips on how to prepare taro, yuca, sweet potatoes and yams, and other root vegetables in chapter ten.

Note: You may want to limit your intake of some of these root vegetables, especially yuca root, if you're suffering from small intestinal bacterial overgrowth (SIBO), have severe gluten sensitivities, or are trying to lose weight.

Low-glycemic fruits

Although most tropical fruit will be off the menu for a while, there are still many others you can enjoy during the elimination phase. Bananas, citrus, avocado, kiwi, and other fruits that have thick, inedible skins are good choices. Although berries are an amazing source of antioxidants and are low in sugar, they can often be contaminated with wild yeast. If you suspect that yeast is a trigger for you, or you continue to flare up during the elimination phase, please consider removing berries from your diet. Washing them thoroughly with a fruit and vegetable wash may make them more tolerable.

Whichever fruits you choose to include in your diet, you will want to limit your number of daily servings to regain insulin sensitivity. If you have been diligent about eating whole, unprocessed foods, haven't been cheating and have been doing your best to keep all trigger foods out of your diet but you're still flaring up, take a long, hard look at your fruit intake. A lot of people really overdo it on fruit and nuts in the beginning, especially dried fruit. Although your body will initially respond fairly well, you'll notice your healing or weight loss hitting a plateau at a certain point if you've got too much of either of these foods in your diet.

MISCELLANEOUS
Coconut butter

Coconut butter is the flesh of the coconut, ground up. It's like any other nut butter (think: peanut butter) and has an amazing flavor. You can make it yourself by chucking a couple cups of unsweetened, shredded coconut into a high-powered blender and turning it on. It can also be purchased online, and even in some progressive grocery stores.

Coconut milk

Coconut milk is a great source of healthy fat. However, when you buy coconut milk from the store it almost always has additives that can be irritating to your gut. Making your own coconut milk is easy; check out chapter ten to find out how.

Coconut flour

Although using coconut flour isn't the same thing as wheat flour, it can be used to bake with. Unfortunately recipes using coconut flour usually call for copious amounts of eggs. You may want to wait until after you've reintroduced eggs to start experimenting with coconut flour.

Coconut water

Coconut water is chock full of nutrients and vitamins, and is often used for electrolytes and to prevent dehydration. (Please note: coconut water does contain sugar. You may want to moderate your intake.)

Black and green pepper, bay leaf, and nutmeg

None of these are nightshades! In fact, studies have shown that these spices help increase tight junction resistance, which may make these non-capsaicin containing spices important in a gut-healing diet.

Hot sauce alternatives

If you miss the spice of peppers and hot sauce, you may be able to tolerate it in small amounts, so test it out on yourself when you're doing your reintroduction. In the meantime, if you're missing the heat, try mustard, wasabi, horseradish, ginger, and black peppercorns.

Fermented Foods

Dairy is off limits during the elimination phase, but you may find that you are able to tolerate yogurt and kefir, as they are gut-nourishing, yeast-free foods. If you cannot tolerate dairy of any kind, there are pretty good quality coconut and almond milk yogurts and kefirs on the market. Be careful, as the cheaper brands are full of stabilizers and added ingredients, including sugar. Look for full-fat, organic options, with no added sugar. There are also heaps of recipes for coconut milk yogurt and kefir available online.

Items to Eliminate First

Your personal triggers will end up being as individual as you are. But until you can zero in on them, you'll need to take them all off the table. In fact, if any of these foods are in your house right now, get rid of them. If they are staring you in the face, it will be hard to say no in a moment of weakness. If you can't bear to throw the junk out, or someone else would be mad at you if you did, move all your healthy stuff together to one place. Chances are this will be the fridge, since you won't be eating a lot of packaged things anymore. And don't forget, this isn't forever. Some of these foods can be reintroduced to your diet if they don't prove to be problematic for you. Let's review these items in greater detail.

ALCOHOL

Sorry to be the one to tell you this, but alcohol can cause leaky gut, and therefore can be a trigger for your HS.

For more than two centuries, alcohol consumption has been linked to increased susceptibility to bacterial infections—especially bacteria that are normally found in your gut. But until recently, no one really knew how gut-derived bacteria were getting into the bloodstream of alcohol users. Thanks to the researchers at the Department of Immunology and Microbiology at the Rush University Medical Center in Chicago, Illinois, we now know that acute alcohol exposure leads to a reduction in the tight junctions between the enterocytes.[29] As discussed back in chapter four, tight junctions fill in the space between the gut's enterocyte cells and, when working properly, prevent the contents of the intestines from entering our bloodstream. Alcohol, however, weakens these junctions, and thus increases your risk for leaky gut and infection.

Though this sort of damage occurs with extreme consumption, you will still need to give up alcohol entirely while your gut heals. Afterward, there's no reason you can't enjoy a drink every so often. Bear in mind, however, that all alcohol contains yeast, some more than others. See page 171. Pure alcohol has been shown to have a limited impact on insulin levels, and moderate drinking can even help improve insulin sensitivity.[30] Just make sure you don't have a sugary mixed drink, or a glass of wine with potatoes au gratin and bread.

CHEMICALS

As discussed earlier, there are two important factors when it comes to intestinal health: the gut barrier and your gut flora. The beneficial bacteria in our intestines help us in all sorts of ways, one of which is maintaining the integrity of the gut wall. For those who don't get the gravity of this, it's important to realize that **more than 70 to 85 percent of your immune system is made up of bacteria that reside in your intestines**. These bacteria are your body's main line of defense against the ravages of the toxic outside world.

Besides creating a leaky gut and ultimately resulting in autoimmune conditions, if your gut flora is compromised, you will get sick—probably quite often. It'll take longer to get over illnesses, they will reoccur, and you will feel like crap. You'll either have diarrhea or be constipated or both, which is never fun.

Chemicals in our environment can destroy our gut flora without our knowledge and may be playing a rather large role in our HS flare-ups. They can also be responsible for recurrent infections.

Chlorine

This isn't much of a surprise: chlorine kills germs—bacteria, viruses, and other microorganisms are totally decimated. There's a reason we put it into swimming pools, and why chlorine bleach is so effective.

Unfortunately, chlorine isn't just in our laundry room or pool—it's also in our tap water. We bathe in it, brush our teeth with it, and drink it. The chlorine in tap water enters our system, either through our mouths or our skin, and kills off the beneficial flora in our guts, our noses, our eyes and our skin. Chlorine doesn't discriminate between good bacteria and bad; it just wipes it all out. Since we know the connection between gut flora health and our immune systems, this doesn't sound like something that we want to have happen.

If it's on your skin, you're basically drinking it so try to make sure that the water you bathe in is as clean as the water you drink.[31] Getting a whole house filter, a reverse osmosis filter for the kitchen, and lowering the temperature of your showers can help. (Our pores open when exposed to warmer temperatures, which allows more chemicals in. Lower temperatures can minimize the absorption.) Try to avoid chlorine pools completely. Salt-water pools are an option.

While you're searching for sources of chlorine in your environment, take a look at the other chemicals you're putting on, in or near your body. Chemicals in lotions, soaps, shampoos, antibacterial creams, and medications can also pose a problem. If you are exposed to chlorine, make sure you take probiotic supplements on a regular basis.

DAIRY

Cow milk was designed for baby cows, so it makes perfect sense that dairy can be very problematic for us in a number of ways. It is possible to be allergic to it, or to have intolerances to either the sugar, or the proteins, in it. Dairy can also cause problems with your hormones, including IGF-1 and insulin. It has been directly linked to autoimmune conditions and certain types of cancer. It most definitely can cause leaky gut. If you are sensitive to dairy, you should see rapid improvement when you remove it from your diet.

The two months I was dairy-free were difficult for me—I eat a lot of cheese and enjoy it immensely. I discovered that slices of avocado can give you the "mouth feel" of cheese and really helps with cravings. Most recipes can be adapted to be cheese-free by simply leaving the cheese out.

Avoid vegan "cheese food." It is made from hydrogenated oils and soy and contains a list of chemicals I can't begin to count, let alone understand. Also avoid the dairy alternatives that contain soy, hemp, and rice. Soymilk should not be consumed as it is made from ... you guessed it, soy. Hemp is a seed. Commercial almond milk and rice milk have practically no nutrition and are full of sugar, artificial vitamins, emulsifiers, and stabilizers. Try making your own nut milk using the recipe in chapter ten. If you find that you are still flaring up after a month on the elimination diet, you may have to give up these milks as they may be a trigger for you. (See Nuts in the *Items to Eliminate Last* section of this chapter.)

Once you've done your initial elimination, try using organic, full fat, raw, grass-fed dairy products during the reintroduction period. If you react to them but still want to eat dairy, the next step is to try goat, sheep, or buffalo products (also organic, also raw). If you react to those, I'm sorry kiddo, you're out of luck. We're just not meant to consume the milk of species other than our own anyway, so chalk it up to your DNA and move on. There is more to life than cheese.

EGGS

Since the lysozyme in egg white sails directly through our gut barrier—and takes other proteins, bacteria, and toxins with it—it can absolutely be a trigger for HS. Although most people find that they are able to reintroduce pastured eggs with little to no problem, conventional supermarket eggs tend to be more challenging. Removing egg whites during the initial elimination phase is highly recommended to allow the gut wall to heal, whether or not eggs end up being a trigger for you. Egg yolks are generally well tolerated and are not associated with leaky gut, but you may want to avoid them during the elimination phase to be on the safe side.

Unfortunately eggs are in most baked goods and a lot of processed foods. Since you will also be avoiding gluten, most of these "foods" will be off the list anyway, but if you're doing your own paleo baking you'll find most recipes call for eggs.

Using arrowroot or even mashed apple or banana in place of eggs is usually pretty effective in baking. Avoid the egg replacer products on the market. In addition to being expensive, they contain gums and starches and usually feature potato starch as their the number one ingredient. Also avoid egg-free vegan products, as they can contain garbage like soy and chemicals and are heavily processed. An egg-free omelet does not exist in nature; nor do egg-free scrambled eggs or egg-free eggs of any kind. I suggest just avoiding eggs altogether during the elimination phase instead of trying to find replacements.

GRAINS, PSEUDO GRAINS & LEGUMES
Wheat and Gluten

We went into great length about gluten in chapter four: it contributes to leaky gut and in recent years wheat and gluten intolerances have become eerily common. In fact, 62 percent of autoimmune patients test positive for wheat intolerance.[5] But get this: In a recent study of HS patients specifically, *100 percent* tested positive.[6] Odds are stacked against you that wheat is a huge problem for you too. And because wheat is also very high in carbohydrates, eating it can easily lead to insulin resistance.

LET'S TALK FIBER

Fiber is very much like a bomb with a time-delay fuse. For a while, it will not visibly affect you, because young people's...intestines are still supple enough to process [it]. Alas, if you keep consuming lots of fiber, your youthful bliss may soon be over. Just ask your parents and grandparents.
— Konstantin Monastyrsky, *Fiber Menace*

I'm really not sure who came up with the idea that human beings need 25-40 grams of fiber a day to be healthy but my gut tells me it was the grain industry. It turns out that all that fiber we've been eating thinking it was good for us actually isn't.

When fiber hits our intestines, it starts to ferment and produce gas. The acidity from the fermentation also causes intestinal inflammation. The combination of the gas and the inflammation causes the intestines to expand just like an air balloon and can cause bloating, abdominal pain, nausea and even vomiting.[7] When fiber—soluble as well as insoluble—reaches the lower intestine, the bacteria go wild, ferment everything in sight and multiply like rabbits. If you don't experience gas after eating fiber, it means that your intestines lack normal bacteria and you are affected by dysbiosis.[8] Until recent technological advancements, fiber wasn't consumed in the large amounts that it is today, as there was simply no way to process it. In fact, the human body lacks the necessary enzyme to fully break it down and digest it, which is why fiber bulks up your stool so much. Some people who try taking fiber supplements in order to "reduce cholesterol levels" even end up developing different digestive disorders.[9]

High fiber diets also increase the elimination of vitamin D3 from our bodies and block the absorption of other important nutrients and minerals. In order to get the recommended amount, you need to consume hundreds of grams of carbohydrates each and every day, which adversely affects insulin levels, hormones, and weight. The fiber you get from fruits and vegetables really is enough to keep you "regular."

Other Grains

All grains contain varying amounts of lectins, phytates, and saponins, which can create leaky gut and lead to HS flare-ups. Although a lot of HS sufferers blame wheat directly for their symptoms, the lectins in grains like corn and even brown rice can also be problematic. These grains also make our bodies produce a lot of insulin, so it's a double whammy. Some grains, like white rice, may be tolerated in small doses; you will have to experiment in the reintroduction phase to see which ones you can have.

Watch Out For: all cereals, wheat, rye, barley, oats, rice, corn, sorghum, millet, spelt, triticale and teff, either in whole form or in flours and starches.

Pseudo Grains and Gluten Free

Pseudo grains such as amaranth, buckwheat, and quinoa are commonly used as grain substitutes in a gluten-free diet. Pseudo grains do contain varying amounts of phytates, lectins, and saponins, which can delay your healing or interfere with other foods you eat. They're also typically high in carbohydrates and can cause leaky gut when consumed in large amounts. Although you may not be sensitive to these items, it is important to remove them during the elimination phase in order to be absolutely sure. Once you've established your triggers, you can reintroduce them to see if they pose a problem for you.

As for trying out some of the new gluten-free foods now on the market, please keep in mind that many GF products contain large amounts of sugar, processed vegetable oils, soy, nightshades, and legumes and can reinforce an addiction. A lot of them also contain potato starch or other things that can be problematic, like rice, tapioca, sorghum, or millet. Making GF items yourself will be your best bet.

Watch Out For: Amaranth, buckwheat, quinoa

Legumes

Legumes are so hard on our digestive system that there are even cute little songs about how much they make us toot. Kidney beans are a personal trigger of mine, and my husband has found that all beans and peanuts aggravate his eczema and IBS. Legumes, like grains, are not part of an ancestral diet unless they've been traditionally prepared. (See page 229 for more information.) They also do a number on our insulin, so you may want to avoid them whether or not they end up being a true trigger for you. Certain legumes like soy also contain phytohormones, which weakly mimic our own hormones. This can cause cascading problems as you are trying to heal.

Watch Out For: Alfalfa, chickpeas, garbanzo beans, fava beans, French and green beans, green and yellow split peas, lentils (all colors), licorice, baby and regular lima beans, mung pea, mung bean, peanuts, kidney beans (all colors), peas (snow, sugar snap, sweet, and green), soybeans

NIGHTSHADES

Cutting out nightshades from your diet can be even more complicated than going gluten free. Ask for tomato-free spaghetti sauce at your local supermarket and the clerk will look at you like you're insane. Most sausages and hot dogs contain some type of nightshade. You can find potato in things like shredded cheese, pesto, and olive oil mayonnaise. Commercial alfredo sauces contain bucket loads of soy and dairy, plus wheat and sometimes even potato. You can order tomato-free pasta sauce online, if you're so inclined, but it often contains things like red peppers. Until you're sure those added ingredients don't affect you, you'll want to make things like sauce yourself. Be sure to check out the Tomato-Free Ketchup in the recipe section of the book. It works well as a pizza sauce too. (Use the Faux-coccia bread recipe in chapter ten for the dough.)

Potatoes

Boil 'em, mash 'em, stick 'em in a stew—potatoes are one of the most versatile foods out there. Let's face it, they taste good and are a comfort food for many of us. Most Western cultures have a traditional potato dish. Italian gnocchi and Polish perogies are made from potato. Even Indian samosas have chunks of potato in them. Then there's potato starch, which we find in all sorts of packaged foods like gluten-free products and shredded cheese (to keep it from clumping). Potatoes in one form or another are in a lot of things.

Unfortunately potatoes contain glycoalkaloids, specifically alpha solanine and alpha chaconine. It's not even controversial whether or not these glycoalkaloids cause leaky gut; for decades, researchers have shown that these substances permeate the gut walls, adversely affect intestinal permeability, and aggravate inflammatory bowel disease.[10, 11]

Exposure to light, physical damage, and age increases the glycoalkaloid content within the potato, with the highest concentrations occurring in the skin and just underneath the skin.[12] To a lesser degree, glycoalkaloids are found throughout the rest of the potato—but still in amounts that may be enough to trigger your HS. While cooking potatoes at high temperatures can partly destroy the toxins, certain cooking methods can actually increase them. For example, peeling and boiling the potatoes will give you the greatest decrease in glycoalkaloids—but deep-frying markedly increases them.[13]

Breeders try to keep glycoalkaloid levels within reasonable limits, but different varieties contain different amounts of the toxins. While a normal potato has 12–20 mg/kg of glycoalkaloid content, a green tuber contains 250–280 mg/kg, and green skin 1500–2200 mg/kg.[14]

PEOPLE OFTEN ASK

me if I miss potatoes. Sure, I miss them. French fries are awesome. Potatoes are versatile and go with everything. They are quick, easy and delicious.

But potatoes make me flare up with boils that take months to go away and leave scars. Boils that are painful, embarrassing, and impact every aspect of my life.

Now, ask me again if I miss them.

There are reports of poisoning and death from eating green potatoes.

Now, unless you're growing the potatoes yourself, by the time you buy them and get them home, they're probably already pretty old. Potatoes are often stored in warehouses for ten to twelve months before they even make it to the inside of a truck. From there, they are battered every step of the way along the long journey to the supermarket, typically averaging hundreds sometimes thousands of miles. Once they reach their destination, they are thrown into a display bin and exposed to light. Remember, the three things that increase the glycoalkaloids in potatoes are age, light, and damage. Check, check, aaaand ... check.

Another interesting thing I found while researching potatoes was the amount and types of inflammatory cytokines that were elevated in the test subjects after consuming potatoes. TNF-α and IL-17 were found to be present in significantly elevated levels.[15] TNF-α and IL-17 are the exact cytokines that are significantly elevated in HS patients.[16,17] I rest my case.

Watch Out For: Potato starch and flour in various baked goods, shredded cheese, and, believe it or not, certain types of condiments like mayonnaise and salad dressing. Potato flour is even used to coat meat for a gluten-free crust at some restaurants and is an ingredient in some sour gummy candies.

Tomatoes

Tomatoes are probably even more pervasive in our culture than potatoes and even more difficult to avoid. Tomatoes are supposed to be healthy. They contain lycopene, a powerful antioxidant that has many health benefits, including protecting your skin from sunburn.

They also contain the potent glycoalkaloids, alpha tomatine and dehydrotomatine. Alpha tomatine is so powerful that it is used in vaccines as an adjuvant[18]—something that's added to the mix to make sure that the recipient actually develops immunity against the virus they are being inoculated against.

The lectin in tomatoes has been proven to pass through the gut wall all by itself. In 1972, a group of researchers fed subjects tomato juice with a radioactive isotopic tracer in it and half an hour later the isotope was in their bloodstream.[19] Although it doesn't cause an inflammatory response on its own like peanut lectin and wheat can, tomato lectin is "sticky" and will bind to other antigens in the gut and bring 'em along for the ride. Curiously enough, alpha tomatine levels in organic tomatoes have been found to be higher than in their conventional counterparts.[20]

Watch Out For: Any product containing tomato. That includes tomato sauce, ketchup, spices, dried tomatoes, green tomatoes

Eggplant

Also known as aubergine and favored by many vegans and vegetarians, eggplant contains alpha solamargine and alpha solasonine, which are steroidal glycoalkaloid derivatives of solasodine. These toxins have been shown to penetrate the placenta in pregnant rats and impact the fetuses. Although the test subjects were fine themselves, their female offspring were shown to have "impaired sexual function" as adults.[21]

The toxins in eggplants also act as phytohormones (plant hormones), meaning they mimic our own hormones. This can create a cascade of problems, as all of our hormones work together in our body to create stability and balance. Throw one of them out of whack and the rest will follow. Solasodine is so powerful it is even used to make some oral contraceptives.

The levels of glycoalkaloids vary in different varieties of eggplants. Wild eggplants usually have more, with some having levels high enough to cause death. Eggplants also contain trace amounts of nicotine.

Watch Out For: Any variety of eggplant; Greek moussaka, some Thai entrees and many Vegan or vegetarian options

Tomatillos

Also known as "husk tomatoes," tomatillos are a curiosity indeed. They are related to tomatoes, but they're not tomatoes. If you're familiar with Latin cuisine, you will probably recognize a tomatillo if you see one. They look like very small tomatoes and are surrounded by an inedible paper-like husk. The fruit itself can be yellow, red, green, or even purple. Tomatillos are a key ingredient in fresh and cooked Latin American sauces, especially salsa verde. Problem is, they are nightshades with a pretty high alkaloid content.

Watch Out For: Tomatillos are often found in Mexican and other Latin cuisines, especially fresh and cooked sauces such as salsa verde

Peppers

Hot peppers contain capsaicin (yet another alkaloid), which is what gives you that burning sensation when you eat them. Although some people enjoy that feeling, it's good to know that large amounts of capsaicin actually increase oxidative stress and can even mess up your DNA. Studies have shown that eating hot peppers releases endorphins (your body's way of dealing with pain), which can result in addiction. Anything that makes us feel good can become an addiction if we're not careful.

Other studies have shown peppers with capsaicin in them increase intestinal permeability as well. In a 1998 study, two different reactions were found; paprika and cayenne pepper not only increased leaky gut, but also affected the ability of the tight junctions to keep other things from leaking out.[22] So, not only will hot peppers give you leaky gut in the first place, they'll increase your leaky gut and make you more sensitive to other things.

Bell or sweet peppers are also members of the *Capsicum annum* family, although they don't have the hotness of their other family members. They are usually treated like a vegetable instead of a spice. They contain less capsaicin than their cousins, but it's still there.

Watch Out For: Sweet or bell pepper (all colors), hot red pepper, chili pepper, cayenne, serrano, jalapeno, paprika, habanero, salsa, spice mixtures, red curry powders, Tabasco sauce, hot sauce, enchilada sauce, and anything hot and spicy. Be wary of brightly colored orange or red food products. Sushi restaurants have been known to add oil of paprika to tuna to make it a brighter color. Paprika extract is often used as a natural color additive in red, pink, and orange candy

Other Nightshades on the Rise

Goji berries are hailed as the greatest thing in antioxidants, but guess what? Yep, they belong to the nightshade family too. Reports of people getting very ill after eating goji berries are littering the Internet. Goji berries contain two novel steroidal alkaloid glycosides called lycioside A and lycioside B. These are found within the seeds.

Another newcomer to the scene is Pepino melon, or melon pear, which is a nightshade and should be avoided. Pimentos and huckleberries, although fairly rare, are also nightshades.

Be careful about taking supplements. Adrenal support supplements can have *ashwagandha* (Indian ginseng) in them—yet another nightshade. Always check the label and if you don't know what something is *make sure you research it before you take it.*

Watch Out For: Goji berries, pepino melon, melon pear, pimentos, huckleberries, and ashwagandha (Indian ginseng)

Tobacco

You may be surprised to learn that the tobacco plant is a nightshade. It contains six different alkaloids: nicotine (which we've all heard of), as well as anabasine, nornicotine, anatabine, cotinine, and myosmine. The amounts vary based on the blend of tobacco and where it came from, but nicotine and nornicotine are usually the two alkaloids that are present in the highest concentration.[32] Although the addictive nature of nicotine is well known, what isn't common knowledge is that all of these other alkaloids have addictive properties and may contribute to a dependency on tobacco.[33]

Many studies have also linked smoking to HS. Whether the tobacco causes the disease or HS patients are so miserable that they turn to smoking remains the issue of some debate—many people with HS have never touched a cigarette. Some sufferers report a lessening of their HS symptoms when they quit smoking. Others (myself included) saw their first HS symptoms appear around the time they first started smoking.

We do know that the connection between tobacco use and gut health has been well studied. Smoking can harm all parts of your digestive system, contributing to common disorders such as heartburn, ulcers, Crohn's disease, and possibly even gallstones. Although we're not entirely sure how smoking causes this damage, some researchers believe that it decreases blood flow to the intestines and causes inflammation."[34]

I believe that tobacco may simply be an explosive kick-start towards developing a leaky gut for individuals who are sensitive to nightshades. When they quit smoking, the damage is still quite extensive and other nightshades, like potatoes and tomatoes, continue the job started by the tobacco.

Since we know the powerful damage that different alkaloids in night-shade plants can cause, it is easy to see that a plant that contains six of them is probably something we want to avoid.

Watch Out For: Cigarettes, snuff and chewing tobacco, secondhand smoke. Nicotine lozenges and gum contain a synthetic form of nicotine that may not be a trigger for you; however, these products often contain sucralose, which may cause a flare-up.

POLYUNSATURATED VEGETABLE OILS

There's nothing natural about industrialized seed and vegetable oils. They are completely man-made. Try turning an ear of corn into a gallon of golden corn oil. You can't—not without chemicals and lots of petroleum. Since these oils are in a completely unnatural state, they don't do us any good when we consume them. Not only do they cause inflammation, they're teeming with lectins, chemical residue, and are usually already rancid by the time they hit the bottle. Our body doesn't recognize them as food and doesn't know what to do with them. Since our system doesn't see these oils as usable fatty acids, the hormone that tells us when we've had enough fat never gets released. This means we can easily eat our way through an entire bag of potato chips, or four helpings of fries, and not be sick to our stomach. (When you start eating animal fat again, you'll see what I mean. You'll only be able to eat about a quarter the amount of sweet potato chips fried in tallow or lard as you would the same chips fried in sunflower oil. In fact, I bet you CAN eat just one.)

Watch Out For: Corn, sunflower, safflower, soy, and canola

PREPACKAGED AND PROCESSED CONVENIENCE FOODS
Sodas (diet or otherwise), store-bought condiments, fast food, frozen dinners, or any other prepackaged and processed convenience foods are off the table. These items often contain gluten, potato starch, yeast, high fructose corn syrup, artificial sweeteners, polyunsaturated vegetable oils, excess salt, food coloring, guar gum, and numerous other stabilizers and chemicals designed to extend a product's shelf life.

SEEDS
Some seeds can be problematic for autoimmune conditions, in particular sesame seeds. Coffee and chocolate are also seeds but most people with HS tend to tolerate them well, so I don't think anyone needs to give them up right away. (See *Items to Eliminate Last*.) As for the other seeds, eliminate them for a month or two during the elimination phase and try reintroducing each type back into your diet and see how they affect you personally.

Watch Out For: Anise, caraway, chia, coriander, cumin, fennel, fenugreek, mustard, nutmeg, poppy, pumpkin, sesame, sunflower, and hemp[23]

SUGAR
I would love to be able to tell you that the occasional binge won't hurt, but I honestly can't. What I can tell you is that sugar is a tricky trigger to avoid. It's addictive, so you'll crave it. A lot of us use sugar for energy, for celebrations, and to reward ourselves—for some of us, it has become our

only friend. But it bears repeating: SUGAR IS NOT OUR FRIEND.

As you can see, a lot of the trigger foods on this list—grains, for example—are converted to sugar in our bodies after we eat them. Then there are the nightshades, which, on top of being high in carbs, contain *glycoalkaloids*, an alkaloid that bonds with a sugar molecule. Even dietary yeast is affected by sugar. If you do nothing else but avoid sugar—and the items that metabolize as sugar—you will definitely come out ahead. And when we talk about sugar, remember that includes fruit juice and high-glycemic fruits. It most especially includes fructose sugar substitutes and high fructose corn syrup, both known to cause metabolic syndrome, obesity, elevated insulin levels, and, yes, HS flare-ups.

Splenda

I used to be a Splenda junkie. I consumed probably half a cup of the stuff a day before I went Primal; it went into my coffee, my baking, on my fruit. I carried it in my purse. I bought prepackaged stuff with Splenda in it. After all, it was "natural," made from sugar. And it was supposed to have no affect on my blood sugar!

Turns out it's the furthest thing from natural that's possible: Splenda contains sucralose, causes weight gain, and it messes up your digestive tract big time.

In 2008, Duke University Medical Center conducted a study that proved that Splenda decimates the good bacteria in your gut, permeates your gut wall, and allows foreign proteins to enter your bloodstream.[24] All this at levels that are less than the FDA approved daily limits. Splenda may very well be YOUR trigger. At the very least, it's contributing to your leaky gut. I have spoken to several women who have had dramatic improvement of their HS once they cut Splenda out of their diet completely.

The authors of the Splenda study state that ingesting the stuff might have "clinical significance for humans in the management of many medical conditions in which gut flora play an important role,"[25] and that it can interfere with many essential gut functions, including nutrient metabolism, normal immune system functioning, gastrointestinal mobility, inhibition of pathogens, vitamin synthesis (B Group and K, and metabolism of drugs.

BLOOD TESTING

A lot of people ask me about getting tested for allergies and intolerances. Even though we've been thoroughly burned in the past, the doctor's office is usually the first place we run to when we're looking for answers. The truth is, in order to find answers in a lab, your doctor is going to have to run expensive tests that are still in their infancy when it comes to accuracy.

Even tests for wheat intolerance aren't accurate most of the time.[42] You may be sensitive to gluten, or gliaden, or WGA, or one of the thousands of other proteins in wheat. Unless your doctor knows what test to request, you could end up wasting your time and money. Blood testing isn't all that accurate anyway. Fecal tests are—but it's incredibly hard to find a doctor that will perform one. (My gastroenterologist actually laughed at me when I requested one.)

Dr. Kenneth Fine at Enterolab developed a test that detects anti-gliaden IgA in stool. He has been performing informal research to see what his fecal test turns out and discovered that the difference in accuracy between the two types of tests is astounding. For example, 57 percent of people who had digestive symptoms tested positive for wheat intolerance by fecal test, whereas only 12 percent of them tested positive by blood. Seventy-six percent of microscopic colitis patients tested positive by fecal test, compared to only 9 percent by blood.

A negative antibody test does not rule out sensitivity to something. It just means that you're not allergic to it. Most of us already know we're not allergic to stuff, but it makes us break out in boils anyway. In my opinion, the best way to test to see if you are intolerant to something, or to see if it triggers your HS, is to eliminate it for thirty days and then reintroduce it.

When I cut Splenda out of my diet, my HS got drastically better and I lost ten pounds without even trying. When I read that sucralose, the main ingredient in Splenda, breaks down into at least fourteen byproducts of chlorine in your body,[26] saying no to it became a lot easier. I didn't know about the other side effects that Splenda had at the time, but I sure reaped the benefits when I quit.

Splenda could very well be another good reason to drink filtered water: a 2011 study found that sucralose is a widespread contaminant of wastewater, surface water, and groundwater in the United States.[27] Rock on.

Honey

Don't include honey in your diet until you've been at this for a while. Although it's natural, it is still sugar. Once your insulin sensitivity returns to normal, you can try small amounts of raw, unfiltered, local honey. Honey is easily digested and contains nutrients and enzymes that can help with allergies. Make sure the honey is local though—you don't need to build immunity to allergies in a place over three thousand miles away. A small amount of honey can help boost energy and help with sugar cravings. If you tolerate it, you can use half stevia and half honey to cut down on the sugar content.

If you're a woman, you may want to avoid honey during the progesterone/testosterone dominant part of your cycle. Too much at the wrong time can contribute to flare-ups.

YEAST

A recent study tested a batch of HS sufferers and found that **100 percent** of them had an intolerance to yeast—brewer's yeast in particular.[28] If you find you react strongly to wheat products, you may very well be reacting not only to the wheat, but also to the yeast itself.

Yeasts are single-celled organisms that are closely related to molds. Both mold and yeast are classified in the kingdom Fungi. People who suffer from yeast intolerance often have environmental allergies or intolerances to molds and fungi as well.

Brewer's yeast and baker's yeast are different strains of the same species of fungi—*Saccharomyces cerevisiae*. (Please note that these strains of yeast are different from candida albicans, which, among other things, causes vaginal yeast infections. If you suffer from yeast infections and HS, you may very well have both an overgrowth of candida and an intolerance to other species of yeast.)

Wild species of *S. cerevisiae* can also be found growing on the exterior of other foods like grains and berries (especially grapes). Dried fruit can cause a flare-up, as can fermented foods such as kombucha, vinegar, and soy sauce. The most common reaction to brewer's yeast is migraines, followed by changes in the skin, including irritation, dryness, itching, and hives.

You may see immediate, painful flares if you consume something that contains both sugar and yeast. That's because yeast feeds on sugar. But unlike sugar, dietary yeast is not always easy to spot, which is why figuring out if yeast is a trigger for you can be frustrating.

Certain foods like beer, wine, bread, and pastries are known sources of yeast and easy to avoid. But some fruits and vegetables are not. You may eat a particular fruit, like berries, many times and have no reaction, because the particular batch you consumed wasn't "infected." However, the next time you buy that same food, it may have yeast or some form of mold growing on it. Thoroughly wash fruits and peel vegetables and you may be able to enjoy them again without the flare-up.

As you go through the following list, bare in mind that there is no way to avoid yeast 100 percent of the time. Mold and fungi are a little easier to spot, but in some form these three types of organisms are often found in many of our favorite foods. If you can limit your exposure you should be in for a pleasant surprise.

A little bit of yeast is not going to slam you directly into Stage III (you may even be able to tolerate a little vinegar from time to time), but knowing which foods are most problematic for you will be a very helpful weapon in your healing arsenal.

Cheese, sour cream, and buttermilk

Quite a few dairy products, including all cheeses, sour cream, buttermilk, and cottage cheese are fermented, and therefore contain live cultures. Unfortunately this means that they may make you flare up; those cultures include yeast and/or fungi, even if they've been pasteurized. Aged and blue cheeses are especially problematic—the blue bits in blue cheese are actually a type of mold called *Penicillium roquefortii* (not to be confused with its cousin *Penicillium chrysogenum*, used to make penicillin). You may be able to tolerate milk, yogurt, kefir, and butter after the elimination phase of the diet. I recommend removing dairy completely. Reintroducing it will be a lengthy process; each type of dairy product must be evaluated on its own.

Baked goods

Foods like pizza dough, bread, bagels, pastry, etc., usually contain wheat, so you will be avoiding these anyway. Still, it's good to read labels and check for baker's yeast. Some gluten-free companies make yeast-free breads; keep in mind if it doesn't say yeast-free on the package, it isn't.

Tea

Most teas (not herbal teas) go through a fermentation process. While this process itself does not involve yeast or mold, the tea may easily become contaminated. Some varieties of tea are purposely aged with natural molds and yeast.

Fermented foods

Anything fermented can contain yeast. This includes kombucha, wine, vinegar, alcohol, soy sauce, cider, and beer. Citric acid, which used to be made from citrus juice, is now made from fermented corn. Other things in this category to watch out for are lactic acid (made from fermented corn or potatoes), MSG (made from the fermentation of sugar or starch), miso, tamari, tempeh, fish sauce, and any preserved or pickled foods. This includes sauerkraut, olives, and pickles. Condiments like olives, horseradish, mayonnaise, ketchup, and mustard often contain vinegar, therefore you need to watch out for them as well.

Watch Out For: Store-bought condiments such as ketchup, mayonnaise, salad dressing, barbeque sauce, prepared mustard, and horseradish. Fermented foods such as kombucha, alcohol, wine, beer, vinegar, soy sauce, cider, miso, tamari, tempeh, fish sauce, and any preserved or pickled foods, including sauerkraut, olives, and pickles. Certain sodas, like ginger ale and root beer (if traditionally prepared) are fermented, as are malt, barley malt, and malted barley flour. Also watch out for almond, vanilla, and other flavor extracts, as they contain alcohol.

NOTE: Fermented foods are extremely healthful and are part of a gut-healing diet. As you reintroduce them, keep your servings small and watch for any change in your skin or digestion. You may be able to tolerate small amounts occasionally, or none at all.

Fruit juices, dried fruit, and unwashed fruit

There are hidden sources of wild yeast in seemingly innocent foods that you need to watch out for. For example, dried fruit can be extremely problematic, especially apricots, figs, and raisins. As previously mentioned, fresh fruits like grapes, blackberries, blueberries, raspberries, and strawberries are often contaminated and can cause a reaction. Jams, jellies, and juices made with these fruits are just as big a problem as the fruit itself. Thoroughly washing the fresh fruit often can alleviate the problem, so it's not necessary to completely cut out berries unless you continue to flare up. Just make sure you clean them thoroughly, and be sure to avoid over-ripe produce altogether.

Canned tomatoes and tomato juice often contain yeast, mold, or both. Besides the fact that tomatoes are a nightshade, high in sugar, and a proven cause of leaky gut, you now have yet another reason to avoid them.

Mushrooms and truffles

It's important to note that fungi of all kinds, such as mushrooms, are relatives of yeast. If you are sensitive to yeast, you may be sensitive to fungi. Truffles, truffle oil, wild mushrooms, dried mushrooms—even mushroom flavoring—may cause a flare-up.

Medications and supplements

Medications like penicillin, amoxicillin, mycin, chloromycetin, and tetracycline are derived from mold. Also, most B vitamin supplements are made from yeast, unless they specifically state otherwise on the package.

> **Watch Out For:** Multivitamins containing B vitamins, tablets made from yeast, and all medications and tinctures containing alcohol.

Peanuts

Peanuts are notorious for being contaminated with mold, yeast, and mycotoxins. A small handful of peanuts can be enough to cause a flare-up.

Yeast spreads and additives

Food spreads like Marmite and Vegemite are nothing but yeast; yeast extract is clearly written on the label, right under the brand name. Also be aware that yeast and yeast extracts are often used in packaged foods as additives or flavorings. Make sure to scan lists of ingredients on any packaged food you buy for the words "aged," "enzymes," "hydrolyzed," "autolyzed," and "yeast." Many companies have replaced MSG with yeast extract, which requires no E-number labeling and can be advertised as "all natural."

Items to Eliminate Last

Although the following items are not usually true triggers for HS, some people report an improvement of symptoms when they're removed from the diet. It may be because the following foods can be contaminated with a trigger—like yeast—or they are being eaten along with a trigger—like sugar—or the individual may simply be intolerant or allergic to them. I suggest eliminating the items we've already discussed, and leaving the next few things for last, unless you've already established they're a problem for you.

COFFEE

Hopefully you won't have to try eliminating coffee unless you've already exhausted all other avenues. Coffee has absolutely no negative effect on me, and if you check out Wendy's story on page 115, you will hear direct testimony from someone who actually did eliminate coffee for over a decade on the advice of a doctor. Removing it had no effect on her—and neither did its reintroduction.

That said, I do know of one person who says that coffee is her trigger. We're all different. Here's hoping that one person is a complete anomaly.

So here's the scoop on coffee beans: they're actually not beans at all. Botanically speaking, they are seeds, the pit from inside the coffee plant's fruit. We only call them beans because they look like them. But they are still seeds and as such, contain lectins, phytates, and other antinutritional factors, which, for the most part, we want to avoid.

Here's the good news: coffee goes through a lengthy processing period before it actually arrives in your cup. First, it's either fermented or it's dried. Fermentation disables some of the antinutrients right from the get-go, but the process requires a lot of water, especially near the end when the beans are thoroughly rinsed. If you're buying coffee that comes from a region where water is scarce, chances are it hasn't been fermented. Drying the beans doesn't do much in terms of disabling phytates, since the beans don't reach very high temperatures at that stage.

Whether it's fermented or dried, the coffee then goes through an (optional) process where the hull is removed and the bean is polished. This process creates lots of friction and heat, makes the bean look nicer, and gets rid of any chaff. The final step is roasting, which destroys most of the beans' phytates,[35] but also destroys any phytase that may be present. (Phytase, the enzyme that neutralizes phytic acid, is destroyed during heat processing.[36])

Any phytates left in the coffee bond with calcium and zinc, and make them unavailable to your body.[37] If you take a zinc supplement, avoid taking it at the same time as your morning cup of joe. You can also make sure that you have lots of beneficial gut flora working for you—they'll produce phytase to help neutralize any phytates which may be left over.

Caffeine is an alkaloid, but it's not from the nightshade family. We don't necessarily need to avoid all alkaloids (they're everywhere, folks), but sensitive individuals may react badly to caffeine. Usually, too much caffeine will make someone nervous, jittery, and anxious or may interfere with sleep. It can cause diarrhea or make people feel sick to their stomachs. If coffee affects you in this way, chances are you have already stopped drinking it. If it doesn't affect you negatively, I seriously doubt that coffee is the source of your HS.

Shade-grown and decaffeinated coffee can contain high amounts of mycotoxins, which can affect, or even cause, leaky gut. Just something to keep in mind when you're at the grocery store.

CHOCOLATE

Chocolate has a very similar back story as coffee; it comes from a seed, contains antinutrients, and goes through a similar, lengthy process before it arrives to the store. Choosing organic dark chocolate (dairy and soy-free) can help to determine whether it's the chocolate—or the additives—that are causing problems.

NUTS

Nuts have been poorly studied for their antinutrient content. Tree nuts (almonds, walnuts, pecans, brazil nuts, etc.) are one of the most allergenic foods out there, however it's unclear if they increase intestinal permeability or adversely affect the immune system.[38]

Unless you are allergic to them, Loren Cordain suggests you try restricting tree nuts last. If, after thirty to sixty days of a strict elimination diet, you are still flaring up, go ahead and cut tree nuts out of your diet and see if it has any effect. You may find that you react specifically to one nut but not to others. You will need to be scientific in your approach if you reach this stage.

Few nuts on the market are actually nuts to begin with: peanuts are legumes and coconuts and cashews are actually fruits. They are *culinary nuts*, meaning that they can be used like real nuts in cooking. Pine nuts, chestnuts, hazelnuts, and acorns are true nuts.

If you do choose to keep a few nuts in your diet during the elimination phase, make sure that they are soaked, sprouted, and roasted to disable as many antinutrients as possible.

You should also be aware that nuts (like seeds) contain high levels of omega-6 fatty acids, which can lead to inflammation—and high levels of inflammation can make HS symptoms worse, so it's good to limit them in any case.

Thankfully there aren't many recipes that absolutely have to have nuts in them. They are fairly easy to avoid and it's usually pretty obvious when they're there. You'll want to check with restaurant staff to make sure they haven't used something like walnut oil in your salad dressing, though, since the concentration of omega-6 is much higher in oil form. Since nut allergies are pretty serious, most restaurants will list it on the menu.

Macadamias, almonds, pecans, walnuts, hazelnuts, and brazil nuts can potentially be problematic, so be on the lookout for them.

THE WHOLE PICTURE

While I was going through this process, I was unwittingly doing other things besides changing my diet that helped. I stopped taking birth control pills and started taking probiotics, vitamin D, zinc, and magnesium. I slept more, exercised properly, avoided alcohol and sugar, and didn't need to take painkillers like Ibuprofen anymore. I started drinking filtered water, stopped eating Splenda and anything artificial, and stopped swimming in chlorinated pools. All these factors, as well as the dietary changes, contributed to my remission from HS. It's important that you read all the information in this book if you want to heal completely. It's not enough to just go gluten free.

SALT

To the best of my knowledge, salt is not a trigger item. But it's worth noting that high salt intake is already a known culprit in heart disease and high blood pressure, and is now being linked to autoimmune disease as well. Researchers have found that adding salt to the diet of mice induced the production of interleukin (IL)-17 T-cells (TH17), cells that have a pivotal role in autoimmune diseases, including HS. Mice genetically engineered to develop a form of multiple sclerosis ended up with a worse form of the disease than mice that weren't given any salt.[39]

Most salt added to processed foods is of the lowest quality possible. It has been stripped of all its nutrients and minerals, bleached and chemically processed. An incredibly large amount of it is used in fast food, to make inferior food taste better. An ancestral diet doesn't contain a lot of salt to begin with, so taking in too much salt shouldn't be an issue. When you do add salt, use a brand that hasn't been bleached and that still contains all its valuable minerals. I like pink Himalayan salt and Redmond's Real Salt. Celtic salt is good too.

What If It Doesn't Work?

If you've been following the elimination diet very carefully and you haven't seen any improvement after thirty to sixty days, there may be other issues at play. You may be experiencing cross-reactivity, during which your immune system confuses the proteins in normally safe foods for proteins that you have an intolerance to. This is very common with wheat or gluten intolerance. A lot of foods can cross-react with gluten, including coffee, soy, chocolate, sesame, and tapioca.[40] Consider removing any of these items that are not already on your elimination diet and see if you get results.

You may also need to try certain fruit and vegetable restrictions if you continue to have digestive issues. Look into Fermentable Oligo-, Di- and Mono-saccharides, and Polyols, also known as FODMAP for short. Foods that contain these forms of carbohydrates can make the symptoms of some digestive disorders, such as irritable bowel syndrome (IBS) and inflammatory bowel disease (IBD), worse. You can find a list of high FODMAP foods in the appendix of this book.

You may also have an overgrowth of bacteria in your small intestine (SIBO), an intestinal parasite, or even a yeast overgrowth that is throwing off your gut flora. You may need to investigate the Selective Carbohydrate Diet (SCD) or look into Gut and Psychology Syndrome (GAPS), both of which are beyond the scope of this book. Getting tested for food intolerances is another option; you may simply still be eating one of your trigger foods, or may be exposed to it in your environment in some way.

If You Absolutely, Positively Can't Handle a Total Elimination Diet

If you are having trouble jumping into an elimination diet with both feet, here's what you can do instead.

First, cut out grains, sugar, and heavily processed foods. Keep at that for a while (at least thirty days) and track your progress. You need to heal your gut somehow, and going gluten-free is the number one step to achieving this. You'll also still need to pay attention to the gut-healing supplements we discussed back in chapter four, *Follow Your Gut*.

Once you've successfully eliminated grains and sugar, begin cutting out other food groups, one at a time: nightshades, dairy, eggs, etc.

Follow all the directions pertaining to the elimination phase, the diet/symptom journal, and reintroduction.

Each food group should be eliminated for at least thirty days, with reintroduction over a period of weeks.

It will be more difficult this way and you may not be able to find a resolution. If you haven't experienced a reduction in the frequency and severity of your flare-ups within a sixty-day period, you'll probably need to bite the bullet and do the full elimination diet.

CHAPTER NINE

Phase II: Reintroduction and Designing Your Personal Ancestral Diet

As you begin to reintroduce and monitor the effects of certain foods, you will gradually move toward a personalized ancestral diet. I want to stress that what you're doing here is making lifestyle changes. This is not a "diet" that you "do" for thirty days, go into remission, and then abandon to return to your old lifestyle habits. In the reintroduction phase, you will begin to experiment as you gradually reintroduce some of the foods you eliminated. You will learn how to make tweaks to your diet that pertain to your individual circumstances.

This is what I call personal science. I assume curious people have been experimenting on themselves for thousands of years. Trusted food sources today were once unknown elements and someone somewhere had to try them first.

Some things we've stumbled on by accident, like beer and clay pots, but it took someone with foresight to realize what they had created and the ingenuity to recreate the exact conditions so they could do it again.

I have been doing little tests to see how I react to certain things since I can remember. When I was younger, these "tests" were more superstitious than they were scientific, but as I've matured, so have my experiments.

Somewhere along the way, we're told that this is the realm of scientists, researchers, and doctors. We may disregard our own findings as irrelevant, because we don't have a degree or a grant.

The truth is, the research these guys are doing doesn't necessarily pertain to you. Just because someone else reacts a certain way to a certain dose of medication doesn't mean that you will too. Personal DNA testing facilities like 23andme.com have shown that genetic variations can cause different drug reactions in different people, and these variations mean that Person A needs a much lower dose than Person B or vice versa.[1] Doctors often prescribe medication doses based on generic findings that don't necessarily work for you.

This holds true of food. We all react slightly differently to the same things. One person may be able to eat wheat with abandon while another ends up in the hospital. If we all follow the USDA dietary guidelines, some of us will end up sick, others fat or diseased, while still others remain perfectly fit and healthy. **It's time to stop being generic and start getting personal**.

Our goal here is to figure out how *you* handle different foods, medications, and environmental factors. Since we can't rely on big studies or doctors to know the answers, we need to use personal science.

Call it self-experimentation, bio-hacking, or N=1—it all amounts to the same thing. You are testing things out on yourself to see how you react.

Dr. Seth Roberts is a personal scientist who works at Tsinghua University in China and at the University of California in Berkeley. When I met him at the Ancestral Health Symposium in 2011, he was discussing the findings of his own personal experiments. He has seen enough evidence over the years to convince himself and others of the value of personal science:

> Personal scientists have big advantages over professional scientists. They have more freedom. They are under no pressure to publish or get grants. They can test any remedy, not just respectable or profitable ones. (American healthcare has been heavily shaped by pharmaceutical research.) Personal scientists are single-minded. They care only about improving their own health, whereas professional scientists have other goals—prestige,

salary, job security, respect of colleagues, and so on—which may interfere with finding the best possible way to improve health. Personal science also benefits from assured relevance. Whatever drug my doctor prescribes, it was developed studying other people. They may not resemble me. The research context (e.g., diet, exercise) may not resemble my life. Personal science studies exactly the person of interest.[2]

The rise of the Internet has made it easier for people to share their findings and to collaborate. Take the information in this book, do some further research online, and start experimenting on yourself. Try to be scientific in your approach and log hypotheses, data, and conclusions. Make a chart if that interests you. Get yourself a lab coat and a pocket protector if that gives you a thrill, and add the term "bio-hacker" to your business cards. If you have any findings of consequence, share them with others. The same things may not work for other people, but by sharing your results, it gives them a place to start.

The most important thing to remember is that the experiments you do on yourself are just as important, if not more so, than the studies you read about in the papers. If you find something to be true for you, then it is. End of story. Don't let anyone tell you that your own intuition and findings aren't relevant just because you can't find them in a medical journal.

And one more thing: keep in mind, I didn't do this all at once—my path to healing really was a journey and it took me several years to get everything locked down. If you're feeling overwhelmed, calm down. Take a look at the list below, pick several things that you believe you can start right away, and just stick to that until you can comfortably do more. This isn't a race. A slow and steady approach will work much better in the long run than sprinting to the finish line.

The Ass-Backwards Plan

When I first went Primal, I cut out all sugar, processed foods, grains, and most starchy carbs, including potatoes. I saw a drastic reduction in the number of flare-ups I had, so much to where I thought I had the HS under control. However, I would break out every so often, seemingly without cause. I followed the 80/20 rule,[3]—that is, striving for 100 percent perfection 80 percent of the time—and for the first year and a half, I treated myself to potatoes, milk chocolate, and even Subway sandwiches once every couple of weeks. Because I wasn't very scientific in my approach and did not keep a diet-symptom journal, it took me three years to really zero in on my triggers. I had cut dairy out to see what would happen and was already gluten-free at this point, but I didn't notice a difference in the HS. It was nice to rule out dairy as a cause, but I still didn't know what was causing the boils or the occasional zit I would get. Up to that point, I had successfully established that wheat and sugar were a problem for me with my other health problems, including PCOS. I was unaware that another food group besides grains, dairy, and legumes could even play a part.

It took me a while to discover nightshades as a major trigger food. What finally tipped me off were my young twin sons who started having eczema and psoriasis outbreaks. They looked like they had third-degree burns on their legs, and their scalps were covered with a yellowish crusty growth that the doctors said was cradle cap. They were two and a half years old! They weren't supposed to have cradle cap anymore, if they were supposed to have it at all. We just couldn't seem to get it under control. We had made sure that they didn't have any wheat or dairy in their diet, but they were still breaking out. They had full-on allergic reactions to tomatoes— red, rosy cheeks, runny noses, and hives. I checked the ingredients in some of their gluten-free products and found potato starch and/or flour in all of them. The kids would scream in pain and claw at their mouths anytime there was chili, hot pepper, or even paprika in their food. I couldn't get them to eat eggplant or bell peppers at all. Then, they suddenly stopped eating potatoes. They just wouldn't touch them.

With a little research, I found out that tomatoes, potatoes, peppers, and eggplants all belonged to the nightshade family. Who would have thought that a potato was in the same "family" as a tomato? We immediately removed any nightshades from the kids' diets. Since I didn't have potatoes or tomatoes in the house anymore, I wasn't eating them either. All of a sudden, I noticed that my HS had gone into long-term remission. Had I kept a food diary, I may have made this connection sooner.

Without keeping a journal, I also overlooked some key information like the cyclical nature of autoimmunity, why my symptoms went into remission sometimes and why the flare-ups migrated to other areas on my body. Without recording what you eat on a daily basis, all of these sort of things appear random. But trust me, nothing is random. There's a reason for everything.

On the Ass-Backwards plan of not recording my diet and symptoms, it took me much longer to recognize that other symptoms presented with my flare-ups. I just hadn't been aware that there possibly could have been a connection between, say, joint pain and HS. Or an itchy scalp and HS, for that matter. I didn't know to look at the bigger picture; my doctors treated each symptom as an individual problem and didn't connect them at all,[4] and I naturally followed suit. When I started tracking all my physical and mental symptoms in relation to food, I started drawing certain conclusions. I found that when I flared-up I also had joint pain, IBS, depression, itchy scalp, ingrown hairs, mysterious rashes, acne, or some other wacky thing going on. These other symptoms tended to resolve much more quickly than the boils, so before the journal I simply hadn't realized that all these problems were related.

I hope my story helps you avoid the same mistakes I made. Let's get going and get you on the right track with journaling your diet and symptoms right now.

Keeping Track

You will want to create some sort of checklist or chart in order to log not only the food you eat each day, but your symptoms as well. Make a note of every physical thing that is going on in your body. In addition to the severity of flare-ups, don't forget to include the following:

- Aching joints or muscles, pain or stiffness, old injuries suddenly "reappearing"
- Itchy skin, including dry skin, rashes, hives, eczema, or dandruff
- Pimples, ingrown hairs, bumps, or spots
- Headaches, migraines, or dizziness
- Congestion, runny nose, or allergy symptoms
- Depression, anxiety, low-mood, or increased stress
- Anything that seems "off": fatigue, insomnia, or waking up tired
- Digestive issues, including upset stomach, gas, acid reflux, bloating, constipation, diarrhea, or changes in bowel habits

Once you have charted your symptoms for a while, you will begin to see connections among what you eat, when you eat it, and how long the symptoms take to come on. My body usually takes about the same amount of time to react to the same foods, so charting the time of day when symptoms appeared was very helpful to me. Including the day of my cycle also helped. I found that I don't react to sugar for the first two weeks of my cycle, but I definitely do in the days leading up to my period.

Your chart will be individual to you, but I use something like the tables featured on these two pages. Feel free to adapt it for your own personal use. There are also journals available for this purpose that are set up and ready to go and even websites that allow you track stuff online. *The Primal Blueprint 90-Day Journal* by Mark Sisson is a great

DATE: WEDNESDAY, AUGUST 15			
CYCLE DAY: 23			
Time	Food	Symptoms	Notes
0000-0400	None		
0400-0800	None	Woke up with boil on chin. Tired, low-mood, moderate joint pain.	From cheese yesterday?
0800-1200	Sausage Bacon Orange Banana Coffee		
1200-1600	Spinach Ham Cheese Grapes Olives	Burping late afternoon, gassy.	
1600-2000	Steak Sweet Potatoes Broccoli Butter	Brief indigestion after dinner	
2000-0000	None		
Following Day: woke up with another boil, on neck			

resource for those of you who like a nice, prepackaged and ready-to-go diet and experimentation journal. (See page 250 in the Resources section for sample pages from Sisson's book.)

Using different symbols or colors can also be helpful for tracking patterns if you don't have a lot of space to write things out in full.

Looking at these entries, what can we conclude? We can *guess* that the dairy at lunch and dinner played a role in the gas, indigestion, and the boil. But to be sure, the same test would have to be run again without the dairy, at least a couple weeks later when the immune system has had a chance to calm down. After recording the results, the test is run again with dairy. By performing repeat tests and recording specific changes, a trend begins to emerge. This is how we zero in on our triggers.

Along the way, you may discover that other foods affect you in different ways that you don't like. For instance, I found out that I had yeast intolerance by tracking symptoms and time. The gas shown in

DATE: SATURDAY, AUGUST 28			
CYCLE DAY: 8			
Time	Food	Symptoms	Notes
0000-0400	N/A		Clear Skin
0400-0800	N/A		
0800-1200	Sausage Bacon Orange Banana Coffee		
1200-1600	Spinach Ham Grapes Olives Coconut Oil	Burping after lunch.	
1600-2000	Steak Sweet Potatoes Broccoli Coconut Oil	GAS!	
2000-0000	None		
Following Day: No Symptoms			

the previous chart could very well be attributed to the grapes at lunch, not the dairy as previously thought. The boil could be the result of the dairy, something in the sausage, or even a combination of the time in your cycle and the grapes. Don't jump to any conclusions without first tracking things for a while.

I know it's complicated. It may help to eat a lot of the same foods at the beginning of the reintroduction phase so that you will quickly learn how you react to them. Chances are, if you've removed sugar and most of the sources of leaky gut, you're going to be feeling a lot better anyway.

Getting Started

Before you start reintroducing foods, it's a good idea to wait until you see some sort of improvement on the elimination diet. There are quite a few factors that determine how long this will take. First off, the sicker you are, the longer it will take to heal. Some will achieve remission in a matter of weeks. Others will get dramatically better but won't achieve complete remission for more than a year as they experiment with different foods and nail down their triggers. Make a goal of thirty to sixty days to really dedicate to making these initial changes, and you'll be able to reassess whether you need more—or less—time in the strict elimination phase as you get closer to the finish line.

You may return to the elimination phase of this program at any time if you need to detox, reduce inflammation, or get rid of trigger cravings. Before you get frustrated with lack of results, be honest with yourself about how out of whack your system is at the moment, how long you've been sick, and how dedicated you've been to the process. Make changes if something isn't working.

I highly recommend that you remain gluten-free, no matter which phase you're in. And you may never be able to reintroduce sugar, nightshades, or yeast. If trigger foods start sneaking back into your diet again, the healing you began to experience with the elimination phase can be reversed. Remember, there is a complicated process your body goes through with autoimmunity—it is way more than just a boil on your butt. Your body had to go through a lot of confusion and damage to produce that boil. Imagine what's going on *inside* your body.

Autoimmune patients often have relapsing and remitting symptoms and can flare up when they have a viral or bacterial infection, are under a great deal of stress, or when they are inflamed.[5] This is something you are going to have to deal with for the rest of your life—it's not going to be cured and go away forever at the end of thirty days.

How to Reintroduce Stuff

Dr. Sarah Ballantyne, a biophysicist and autoimmunity expert, says that when you reintroduce a food, eat a very small amount of it at least twice on two consecutive days.[6] She suggests waiting at least three days in between different foods, but I would go even further and suggest you wait one full week—HS boils can take their time to appear. If you do have a violent reaction, you will have to wait a couple of weeks for your immune system to calm down before reintroducing any other food.[7]

During reintroduction, it's important that you give each food a fair chance to wreak havoc (or not) before you move on. Here's a rundown of the process. Please note: **You should stop the experiment at the first sign of any of the symptoms listed on page 184.** If any of these symptoms occur, it means you are reacting to the food and it is currently not *GRAS* (generally regarded as safe) for you. Once you've successfully gone a week without any type of reaction, you can consider that particular food to be GRAS and add it back into your diet.

- **Day One:** Eat a very small amount of potential trigger.
- **Day Two:** Eat a small amount of same trigger.
- **Day Three:** Eat a moderate helping.
- **Day Four:** Make it the focus of a meal.
- **Day Five:** Take the day off—no potential triggers.
- **Day Six:** Take the day off—no potential triggers.
- **Day Seven:** If no symptoms, assume the food is GRAS. If you experienced symptoms, the food is not GRAS.

Sometimes, we can tolerate small amounts of our triggers before we flare up. I find this particularly true of yeast, which is why I suggest making the potential trigger food the focus of a meal on day four. If you do not react to the very small amounts of the food the first two days, it's a good idea to see how much of the trigger your body can handle. Do this by increasing the amount of the food you eat over the first four days. It's also important that you return to a trigger-free diet on days five and six. Three days seems to be the magic number for symptoms (especially gastrointestinal) to manifest and resolve, so if that big meal was what tipped your immune system over the edge, you'll know by day six. If you haven't experienced any symptoms by day seven, you can assume you're good to go and can reintroduce another food.

Make sure you add foods back one at a time. Do this slowly. If you introduce different foods less than a week apart, you won't be able to tell what is or isn't affecting you. For me, flare-ups appear the following morning after I have eaten a trigger food. Flare-ups caused by yeast can take three or four days to manifest. It may be different for you, depending on how insulin sensitive you are, how leaky your gut is, how long you've been healing, how much of the food you consumed, and what it was that you ate.

You may want to spend a couple weeks combining different foods to see if you react to them together. For example, the

FINDING YOUR OWN PLAN

Whichever changes you choose to adopt, you're going to have to make this "diet" your own, eventually. Every person reacts differently to different things. You may find you're able to eat some foods that others can't, like rice. You may not be willing or need to give up dairy or eggs. Your diet will become as individual as you are. Once you've been experimenting with eliminations, you'll get a better feel for what your body will allow you to eat. Check out the recipes at the back of this book when you first start out. I also post new autoimmune recipes on my website all the time and the Internet is loaded with them. You'll soon come up with other dishes that you and your family love. I suggest creating a recipe book with all your new favorites so you have them in one place.

saponins in quinoa may increase your reaction to other potential triggers, such as mushrooms. You may be able to handle mushrooms in small doses, but when combined with a saponin- or lectin-rich food, they can become a violent trigger. Eggs too; you may be able to eat something like dairy on its own, but pair it with eggs and you could have a reaction. Remember, saponins, lectins, and lysozyme can cross mucous membranes and bring along other toxins for the ride.

Pay attention to other signals your body is sending you besides the HS. For example, if you eat tomatoes and immediately have joint pain, make a note. If the joint pain subsides on day two, but you have an HS flare-up on day three, the joint pain may have been an early indicator that your body was experiencing inflammation and launching an autoimmune response. It just took a couple days to manifest as HS.

Also bear in mind that there is a clear connection between inflammation and autoimmune disease. Anything that causes inflammation, like insulin and sugar, will likely be problematic for you. The problem is, sugar usually won't make you flare up the first time you have it. It's when you've eaten it for three or four days in a row that you're going to start having problems. (I don't recommend reintroducing sugar in the first place. Instead, try to have sweets only on special occasions—sugar makes autoimmune conditions worse over time.)

After a couple of months, you should have a fairly good idea of many of your triggers. You may find you no longer have to keep track religiously of what you eat. Eating similar foods from day-to-day can help with this. If you tend to eat the same things and only mix it up from time to time, it will be obvious when something "new" is a problem.

Once you have found the foods that are giving you grief, don't eat them anymore, unless the short-term gain caused by that food outweighs the weeks of pain from an outbreak. Sometimes it may. Most of the time, it won't. Let's be honest, your mom's spaghetti and meatballs is good, but is it *that* good?

You may find the boils heal faster if you have your trigger foods only occasionally, or you may find that you now react even more violently than before. Everyone is different; you need to find out how you react.

Once you have a good idea of your triggers, test out your theory by abstaining from them for a while and then reintroduce them down the road when your immune system has calmed down. Did you flare up? How many days of eating that food did it take for you to flare up? Was it all just a cosmic coincidence? If you react again, you have your answer.

What to Reintroduce First

Sarah Ballantyne has classified foods from lowest to highest likelihood to be problematic for autoimmunity on her website PaleoMom.com. I've included this list so that you have a good place to start. If you've previously identified any of these foods as being a trigger for you, or

Least likely to be a problem
Egg yolk (from soy-free, wheat-free pastured chickens)
Ghee (from grass fed dairy)
Seed-based spices (as long as they're not from nightshades)
Starchy vegetables (except tapioca/cassava/yuca)
FODMAP fruits and vegetables (if you've been avoiding them)
Next Least Likely to be a problem
Seeds (except sesame seeds)
Nuts
Alcohol (in small amounts)
Grass-fed butter
Moderately Likely to be a problem
Eggplant and sweet peppers
Paprika
Coffee
Cocoa/chocolate
Sesame seeds
Tapioca/cassava/yuca
Yeast
Grass-fed raw cream
Fermented grass-fed dairy
Most Likely to be a problem
Egg white
Chili peppers
Alcohol (in large quantities)
May Always be a problem
Tomatoes
Nonsteroidal anti-inflammatory drugs (NSAIDs)

Based on Problematic Foods In Autoimmune Conditions by Dr. Sarah Ballantyne, BSc, PhD (2012) if you've had food sensitivity testing done and they've popped up, just leave them out.

I suggest starting with the least problematic foods first and work your way down the list. You'll notice that all the foods on this list are normally consumed on a regular Primal or Paleolithic-style diet. Things like wheat, sugar, potatoes, soy, and other legumes are not ancestral foods, and should therefore not be reintroduced into your diet. (I personally struggle to call any of these things "food.")

As you continue with reintroduction, you'll have some setbacks, some flare-ups, and some moments when you are so tempted to cheat that it hurts. You should notice that those setbacks and flare-ups aren't as bad as they used to be, and those cravings will subside—I promise. Use the strength within you—that same strength that got you through the HS and all those doctors' appointments—and you will eventually come out on the other side healthier, happier, and HS-free.

Whoops, I Flared Up Again

Accidental Dosing

My friends love it when I refer to inadvertently eating bad stuff as "being dosed." Honestly, anytime someone puts poison in my food without me knowing, I consider it a violation. It's like I've been slipped a drug.

Case in point: dining out. I hate to be the one to break this to you, but the restaurant industry is not your friend. Practices common at restaurants can inadvertently make you flare up, even if you think you're choosing the safest option on the menu.

Let's say you go to a steakhouse with friends for a celebratory dinner. You choose a huge steak, with sweet potato fries and steamed broccoli. You put lots of butter on the broccoli, because you've already done testing on dairy and it doesn't affect you. You eat it all. It tastes great.

The next morning, you wake up with a huge boil. What happened? You were so careful! You didn't even have any wine with dinner and you skipped dessert! This is so unfair. It must have been stress that caused the flare-up. Better hit the gym.

Hold on, hold on. Let's rewind to last night and see just exactly what could have happened to cause this.

The steak that you ordered didn't have anything on it. You even asked them to hold the sauce. What you didn't know is that that steak was high in omega-6, because it came from a corn-fed cow, who was also pumped full of antibiotics. Once the meat got to the kitchen, it was marinated in ... something. Perhaps that "something" had soy sauce or hot peppers in it. It may have been some tenderizing concoction full of gluten and chemicals. Regardless, once it was marinated, it was brushed with a gluten-solution to make those beautiful char-marks. That's right, it wasn't the barbecue that made those marks. It was gluten.

I DON'T ADVOCATE

reintroducing gluten, ever. It's an inflammatory protein at the best of times, and if you have a condition like hypothyroidism and possibly an autoimmune disease, it's not a good idea. Corn is a common cross reactant to gluten, meaning that if you're sensitive to gluten, you will often be sensitive to corn. Nightshades and dairy are more individual.

—Chris Kresser, L.Ac,
November 2011

Let's take a look at your sweet potato fries. You think that the chefs are in the kitchen lovingly peeling whole sweet potatoes? Ha ha ha, think again. They opened up a package and dumped them in the fryer. If you lean in close, you can just make out the ingredients on the package in the trash can:

Sweet potatoes, canola oil, modified food starch, wheat flour, tapioca dextrin, salt, sugar leavening (sodium acid pyrophosphate, sodium bicarbonate), xantham gum, paprika extract, sodium acid pyrophosphate.

Modified food starch can come from anything, including corn, wheat, and potatoes. The rest of the ingredients are a mess of triggers and gut irritants. What about the oil they fried your sweet potato fries in? Soy oil, more than likely, but it could have been corn. They also fried a lot of other things in that oil before you got your meal, including onion rings, regular French fries and breaded meat.

Steamed broccoli ... we should be safe here, right? Nope. That broccoli was steamed, all right, and then a mixture of "spices" was added to it. Those spices sometimes contain MSG, yeast, gluten, sugar, nightshades, and more salt. And the butter you added to the broccoli? It wasn't real butter. Oh, I know the waitress said it was butter (well, she *called* it butter), but it was actually a mixture of half butter and half margarine. Margarine made with hydrogenated soy, corn, and canola oil. Yum-O.

Now that you know what you really ate for dinner last night, can you really blame that boil on stress?

Eating out at restaurants is an almost impossible task for me if I want to stay in remission. For a while, I only ate at sushi restaurants. I "cheated" with rice until I found out that they added sugar to it. I "cheated" with California rolls until I read the ingredients on a package of imitation crab:

Alaska Pollock, Water, Egg Whites, Wheat Starch, Sugar, Corn Starch, Potato Starch, Sorbitol, Contains 2 percent or Less of the Following: King Crab Meat, Natural and Artificial Flavor, Extracts of Crab, Oyster, Scallop, Lobster and Fish (Salmon, Anchovy, Bonito, Cutlassfish), Refined Fish Oil (Adds a Trivial Amount of Fat) (Anchovy, Sardine), Rice Wine (Rice, Water, Koji, Yeast, Salt), Sea Salt, Modified Tapioca Starch, Carrageenan, Yam Flour, Hydrolyzed Soy, Corn, and Wheat Proteins, Potassium Chloride, Disodium Inosinate and Guanylate, Sodium Pyrophosphate, Carmine, Paprika.

I underlined all the potential triggers for you. I also underlined carmine, because it's a brilliant red food coloring made from crushed up insect shells. Mmmmm ... I especially love how they have to let us know that the refined fish oil adds a trivial amount of fat. If it weren't refined, it would be the healthiest thing in there.

All jokes and brilliant investigating aside, do you know what else is in that California roll? I don't. There's some sort of sauce mixed in with the "crab." There's sugar in the rice. There's gluten in the soy sauce. Artificial colors, chemicals, and starch in the wasabi. Other than that, we should be safe, but come on! Restaurants are out to make a buck. Employees often don't know what's in the food, as many of the items on the menu are not prepared in the kitchen with fresh ingredients. Too often, the food arrives to the kitchen precooked, frozen, and vacuumed packed. Your server can't make substitutions or leave things out because machines in places far, far away have already prepared the meal.

This is why I prepare my own food. That way, I know exactly what

I am eating. If you choose to eat out, I would love to suggest small mom-n-pop joints, but even then, you have no guarantee that these establishments aren't using cheap ingredients to cut costs. Large chain restaurants are even worse. Cheese is not cheese; it's modified food starch with casein and "cheese" flavoring. Butter is not butter; it's hydrogenated soy oil. Salad dressing contains wheat, soy, corn, dairy, and is loaded with chemicals. It all makes me sick—literally and figuratively.

What I can suggest is eating at a place that offers a gluten-free menu. Tell the waitstaff that you are allergic to soy, wheat, corn, tomato, and potato and see what is left on the menu to choose from. You'll be amazed at what innocent looking options are suddenly no longer available to you, once you feign an allergy and expose the hidden ingredients.

READING LABELS

You'll definitely want to do your research before you set foot in a grocery store. Labeling can be so misleading that you think you are buying something good for you, only to come home and find out that it has fifteen different types of garbage in it. Buying food that doesn't have any packaging at all—whole, unprocessed, organic foods—takes the guesswork out of the equation. But if you do decide to add packaged foods back into your diet, Jayson and Mira Calton's book *Rich Food, Poor Food* is an excellent resource to help you navigate the grocery store and pick the best products out of a sea of prepackaged crap.

You can also bring certain ingredients with you. The staff at seafood restaurants may snicker behind my back when I bring grass-fed butter, a tea light warmer to melt it, and Primal biscuits along with me, but I don't have to worry about hidden ingredients or saying no to the bread. Carrying ingredients like stevia, gluten-free tamari, olive oil, and coconut oil in your purse is always an option; you never know when it will come in handy.

Healing From an Accidental Dosing

If you're healthy and don't have celiac or gluten sensitivity, the damage to your enterocytes from a single dose of wheat heals pretty fast—it takes anywhere from a few days to a few weeks. You may be asymptomatic during most of that time.[8] If you have gluten sensitivity, celiac, uncontrolled inflammation in the gut, nutritional deficiencies, gut dysbiosis, infections, stress, body-wide inflammation or chronically elevated insulin, healing is going to be much slower.[9]

If you're exposed to one of your trigger foods, it can take weeks for your immune system to settle down. Be extra careful (especially with sugar) during that time and let yourself heal. From that point on, pay extra close attention when you're eating things that other people (or machines) have made.

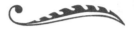

CHAPTER TEN

PrimalGirl Recipes

Changing your diet can be difficult, especially if you're used to opening a bag, can, or box whenever you feel like having a snack. You'll now be cooking with whole foods, monitoring each ingredient that goes into your mouth. To be sure, eating this way requires a lot of dedication and planning ahead, not to mention additional time in the kitchen. Try to see this in a positive light if you don't already. After all, you will be preparing nourishing autoimmune Primal/paleo foods that will heal your body and make you feel great.

If you don't know how to cook, you're not alone. This was something previous generations learned from their parents. Now, many of our parents don't know how to cook, either. Some people can't even figure out how to turn on an oven, much less sauté a few veggies. This is one of the many by-products of our modern culture.

We lead busy lives these days. Many of us have full-time jobs, care for children, clean the house ... all while trying to maintain some level of sanity. For many, microwaving a frozen meal, picking up dinner at the supermarket deli, or dining out has become the new normal.

PREPARING YOUR OWN

food can be empowering, if you let it. With the right attitude, the kitchen can be a place to reflect, discover, and connect. Consider the following suggestions.

Happy people do things with their hands—cooking can be your "thing" for a while.

Engage your senses and touch the ingredients, feel their texture, and discover what real food smells like.

Learn what to do with all those weird kitchen tools.

Spend some quality time with a friend or significant other and recruit him or her into the kitchen to prepare a meal you will enjoy together.

Spend some quality time by yourself and play some energizing music while you dance around the kitchen.

If all else fails, drag your laptop into the kitchen and turn on your favorite soap opera or reality show. Or better yet, get caught up on your reading and listen to an audiobook.

But think about this: throughout human history, up until relatively recently, we spent most of our day in search of food. It's one of our most basic needs, right up there with securing shelter. If we don't eat, we die. Yet in our modern society, that very basic, life-sustaining task of hunting or gathering the food that fuels and nourishes our bodies has become a mere afterthought. We've given up that power to large corporations that care more about bottom-line profits than our best interest.

I simply can't stress this enough: food is extremely important when it comes to our health. Yet many people don't get this very basic principle. I've corresponded with numerous individuals who don't trust that they have the willpower to change their diet to the extreme that it takes to put their HS into remission. They go "all in" for a while, and then fall off the wagon. Before they know it, they're picking up fast food for dinner and their HS flares up worse than ever.

It really doesn't matter how good those french fries taste, how little time you have, or how little money you make. If you choose to eat a standard American diet (SAD), your HS will continue to be a problem. Ultimately the power to end the pain lies with you and the choices you make.

Taking the time and knowing exactly what you put into your body—and into the mouths of your children and pets, for that matter—can provide a sense of satisfaction that mindlessly breezing through a drive-thru never will. When you cook your own foods, you have control over every ingredient that passes beyond your lips. Plus, you gain insight into how your body reacts to each one of those ingredients. Compare that to the fifty-six different ingredients in your sad SAD lunch.

So if you don't know how to cook, it's time to learn. Enroll in a basic cooking class. Research what to do with various whole foods online. Learn from friends who have a handle on navigating the kitchen. Ask one of your gourmand friends to show you how to turn on the stove. While you're at it, ask them what "sauté" means and what that kitchen tool that looks like a porcupine—the one your mother-in-law gave you as a wedding gift—is supposed to do. And for the sake of all that is good and decent, learn to cook like your grandmother did.

Grandma likely didn't follow recipes most of the time. She probably had the skills to know when meat was cooked simply by touching it. She could throw a bunch of leftovers together and somehow it always worked out. Taking an actual cooking class can help you learn these skills if you weren't lucky enough to have them passed down to you. If not a cooking class, consider buying a book on basic cooking techniques, streaming a cooking video, or even checking out how to poach albacore tuna on YouTube. (It's amazing what you can learn in three minutes! And while you're there, plug "autoimmune paleo recipes" into the YouTube search field and find a load of fresh, new ideas to try.)

Here's another tip: cook ahead. My friend Orleatha cooks for an entire month in one weekend—she calls it batch cooking. I tried this and it ended up taking me about a week, but with more practice and planning, I could have made it faster. In reality, the food I make in any given month ends up lasting longer than a month. Most of the time I have ready-to-go meals at my fingertips. Here's what I do:

For an entire week, I don't just make dinner: I make four dinners. Four times the amount that I know my family will eat. After dinner, I then portion out the remaining food in separate containers and freeze them for later. Sure, you spend a lot of time in the kitchen one week out of the month, but you have the rest of the month off.

Due to the incredible amount of planning and preparation it takes to do batch cooking, you may want to check out BatchCookery.com, where Orleatha has put together a program to help you prepare recipes, grocery shopping lists, and maximize your time in the kitchen. She is able to make forty meals for a family of four (160 servings) in fewer than six hours—but there is a lot of planning ahead involved.

Planning ahead also works for breakfast and lunch. If you're not sure what to take to work tomorrow, why not make extra and take tonight's leftovers? There's no rule that says you can't have leftover stir-fry for breakfast.

Stocking your pantry properly will help you to quickly and easily prepare meals and snacks. If you have most, if not all, of the ingredients featured on page 230 in your kitchen, you'll be able to make most of the recipes in this book without having to leave the house.

Essential Tools and Equipment

Slow cooker

This is one of my favorite tools to use, since I can set it and forget it. Recipes like bone broth can literally be left on low heat for days and you don't need to worry about the house burning down. I love waking up in the morning to the smell of baked apples and cinnamon wafting up the stairs, after I've made applesauce the night before. Some people I know actually take their slow cookers with them on vacation. It's nice to have dinner waiting for you in your hotel room, after a long day of sightseeing and exploring.

As you experiment with different cooking techniques, you'll come to appreciate the depth of flavor that a slow cooker can add to your dishes. Low and slow is the rule here.

Marinating meat, herbs, and vegetables in a Ziploc bag and storing them in the freezer until you're ready to use them can be handy when you've got a slow cooker; simply remove the bag, place the food in the slow cooker, and turn it on. Increase the cooking time by several hours, or even double it, if cooking from frozen.

Vitamix blender

This is a big investment. I struggled with spending over $400 on a blender—and it took me over a year to actually buy it—but I have never once regretted the purchase. Cheaper, lower-powered blenders just can't do what the Vitamix can. It makes coconut butter in under two minutes, coconut and almond milk in under five, various nut butters, and probiotic smoothies easily. I can add the entire fruit or vegetable to a recipe. Compare that to fiber-less, sugar-laden juices!

Many paleo baking recipes, like pancakes and cookies, turn out better when they've been whipped in a Vitamix first. I made baby food in the Vitamix and got a fine, smooth texture—even when meat was involved.

When you purchase a Vitamix, you'll also get a dry container, which is ideal for making your own flour. I make sweet potato, yam, and plantain flour by first peeling, then thinly slicing the fresh tuber, dehydrating the slices, and finally, giving them a whirl in the Vitamix dry container. You can use this flour to make baked goods, pasta, and more.

Mandolin and spiral slicer
A sharp mandolin slicer makes uniform slices thinner than a knife ever could, making treats like homemade sweet potato chips easy and accessible—as long as you've got the right fat to fry them in. A mandolin slicer makes easy work of slicing a lot of vegetables at once, for example if you're canning or preserving something, or making your own baby food. Spiral vegetable slicers, like the Paderno World Cuisine Tri-blade, can make boring vegetables fun again. I use the spiral slicer to create quick and easy zucchini noodles, hash-browned sweet potatoes, and interesting salads.

A few good knives
You're going to be cutting up a lot of vegetables, tubers, meat, bones, and other interesting new things as you embark upon this new lifestyle so you'll need to invest in a few good knives. A chef's knife is particularly useful and versatile; you'll also want a small paring knife for peeling, and a serrated knife for cutting up smooth or slippery stuff. Other gadgets worth your time are a knife sharpener, a wooden cutting board, a pair of kitchen shears, and a cleaver to cut through bones.

Deep freezer
This lifestyle becomes progressively easier to follow when you have sufficient storage space to plan ahead and make things in advance. Getting an extra freezer will give you much needed space to store extra broth, tallow, grass-fed steaks from your cow share, healthy homemade popsicles, and whatever else. If you don't have enough freezer space, you may find yourself passing up great opportunities on bulk items.

A Costco membership

While I don't want to advertise for one particular box store, I have to give Costco credit where it's due. They have significantly increased the amount of organic and grass-fed products they carry, and even stock hard to find items like coconut oil and avocado oil. I buy grass-fed butter and cheese, organic almond butter, nitrate-free bacon, sausage, and turkey breast, and even organic salad mixes at Costco. They don't have everything, but they carry enough of my favorite staples that I can do the majority of my shopping there.

The Recipes

The recipes in this chapter are laid out in two parts: *PrimalGirl Basics: Day One and Beyond* is designed for everyone at any phase of recovery. They are void of both gut-irritating Neolithic foods and common HS trigger foods. I encourage you to add them to your recipe collection when you enter the elimination phase, and continue to use them as you transition into your personalized ancestral diet. I further encourage you to explore the wide array of paleo cookbooks on the market as well as all the great recipes featured on Primal/paleo-friendly websites. (See the Resources section in the back of the book for recommendations.)

In *Building Your Personalized Recipe Collection*, you'll find Primal friendly recipes (low-carb, low-sugar, and no gluten, grains, or legumes) that are free of *most* HS trigger foods but may contain a single ingredient—like yeast, eggs, or dairy—to experiment with. Any potential trigger food is indicated in each recipe with a symbol, so you can easily see what's available to you. Once you've established your personal trigger foods during the reintroduction phase, you can include these recipes in your personalized collection, make small changes, or ditch them altogether.

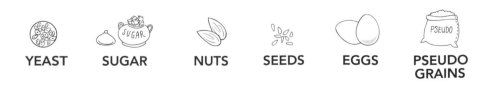

YEAST   SUGAR   NUTS   SEEDS   EGGS   PSEUDO
                                                 GRAINS

PrimalGirl Basics: Day One and Beyond

COFFEE AND "CREAM"

MAKES 1 SERVING

If you absolutely have to have cream in your coffee, you'll be pleased to know that you don't have to give it up. Coconut cream and coconut milk are a couple of creamy alternatives to traditional creamer. Many in the paleosphere love this option. But if you're like me and don't much care for the flavor, try using coconut oil instead. You'll need a blender for this one, since you'll be left with a greasy oil slick on top of black coffee if you use just a spoon.

  1 cup black coffee
  1–2 tablespoons coconut oil or grass-fed ghee

Blend both ingredients on high in blender, until the coffee turns a cream color. Sweeten with stevia if desired. Enjoy hot.

BACON MAPLE LATTES

MAKES 1 SERVING

  1 cup black coffee
  1–2 tablespoons bacon fat
  1 tablespoon coconut oil or ghee
  Maple syrup to taste (optional)
  Crumbled bacon (optional)

Blend coffee, bacon fat, and maple syrup on high speed until coffee is a cream color. Sprinkle bacon on top. It's like a pancake breakfast in a cup.

BONE BROTH
MAKES 8–12 SERVINGS

This recipe requires a slow cooker, and is simple and fairly hands off. You can start with an entire chicken and remove the meat after several hours, then add the bones back in to continue cooking. Or you can just use the left over bones from a baked chicken. You can also save the bones in the freezer until you are ready to use them. Be sure to use a pasture-raised chicken or turkey for this recipe.

Bones of an entire chicken or turkey, chopped so they fit in the pot
Chicken or turkey neck, organ meats, or extra bones
Chicken feet, for extra thick broth
1 onion, roughly chopped
2–3 celery ribs, roughly chopped
2–3 carrots, roughly chopped
2–3 garlic cloves, more if you really like garlic.
1 bay leaf
2–3 tablespoons lemon juice (use apple cider vinegar if yeast is
   not an issue)
Salt to taste

1. Combine all ingredients in a crockpot and cook on low for 12 to 48 hours, depending on how rich you like your broth.
2. After slow cooking, turn off crockpot and let cool until you can work with it
3. Remove and discard bones, vegetables, and other solid matter.
4. Add salt to taste.
5. Strain broth through a clean cotton tea towel into mason jars (a funnel works well for this step).
6. Refrigerate until fat forms on the top. Remove fat (if desired). Do not discard gelatin.
7. Store in the fridge or the freezer until you're ready to use it. Will keep in the fridge for several days. I freeze mine and keep at room temperature for several hours to defrost.

COCONUT MILK

MAKES 4 CUPS

You'll want to get a tea towel, a clean glass bottle, and a funnel ready for this recipe, as well as your blender.

1 cup unsweetened coconut (flaked, shredded, raw, etc.)*
4 cups filtered water, boiling
Pinch of salt
1 teaspoon gluten-free, alcohol-free vanilla, optional
1 teaspoon sweetener (honey, sugar) or ½ teaspoon liquid stevia, optional

*You may increase this up to two cups for thicker milk.

1. Place the coconut in your blender, and add the boiling water. Pulse to mix the two together. Let the coconut soak until it starts to soften, approximately five minutes.
2. When you're ready, turn the blender on high for approximately 2–3 minutes. Turn off and allow milk to cool until you are able to handle it.
3. Set up your glass bottle, funnel, and tea towel.
4. Pour the coconut milk through the tea towel and the funnel into the bottle. When all the liquid has passed through the funnel, squeeze the cloth into the bottle to release the rest of the milk. You can discard the leftover pulp or save it for recipes. Repeat until all the milk is strained.
5. If desired, return milk to the blender, add vanilla, salt, and sweetener, pulse to mix, and enjoy.

Will keep in the fridge for three to four days. Shake vigorously to mix before using. Can also be frozen, but be prepared for some separation when it thaws.

Nut milk version: You can use this exact same recipe to make cashew milk, almond milk, or any type of nut milk, including a wonderful blend of all your favorites. Just make sure you soak, drain, and rinse the nuts first and use fresh, filtered water in your recipe.

COCONUT CREAM
MAKES ABOUT 12 OUNCES

Mickey Trescott, the author of *The Autoimmune Paleo Cookbook*, uses coconut cream to get a rich, creamy flavor in her recipes. She says that although you can buy it premade in the store, it is much more cost-effective to make it yourself. I suggest using a high-powered blender such as a Vitamix for this recipe. Coconut cream can be used to make mayo, caesar salad, or ranch dressing, and can be added to sauces and curries. It is also sometimes referred to as coconut butter.

4 cups dried, unsweetened coconut flakes
Sea salt to taste

1. Place the coconut flakes in a high-powered food processor or blender.
2. Process on high speed, while scraping down the sides with a tamper (you may have to stop and do this manually if you are using a food processor). Process for about a minute at a time, taking breaks as to not overheat the motor. After about 5–10 minutes, you should be left with a smooth, creamy liquid.
3. Place in a glass jar and keep at room temperature.

Reprinted with permission by Mickey Trescott, The Autoimmune Paleo Cookbook, *2013.*

GARLIC "MAYO"

MAKES 12 OUNCES

While it's not going to be as thick as regular mayonnaise made with eggs, this mayo-substitute is creamy and autoimmune friendly. Add some lemon juice and seasonings, and turn it into salad dressing.

½ cup coconut cream (page 206), slightly warmed
½ cup warm filtered water
¼ cup extra-virgin olive oil
3–4 garlic cloves
¼ teaspoon salt

1. Place the coconut cream, warm water, olive oil, garlic cloves, and salt in a blender and blend on high for a minute or two, until the sauce thickens.
2. Let cool for an hour at room temperature. Alternately, you can place it in the refrigerator for 20 minutes. If you would like to use the sauce in a cold dish, thin with water until the desired consistency is reached.

Note: Keeps well in the refrigerator, but hardens. Let it come to room temperature or warm gently before using.

Reprinted with permission by Mickey Trescott, The Autoimmune Paleo Cookbook, *2013.*

TOMATO-FREE MARINARA SAUCE
MAKES 6–8 SERVINGS (1/2 CUP EACH)

This recipe can be used for many things: pasta, casseroles, pizza, chili, or anywhere you would like a tomato-based sauce. It tastes pretty close to tomato and is great poured over spinach or zucchini "noodles." The beets are mostly just there for color. If I have fresh or frozen cranberries on hand, I'll throw in about a cup for extra tartness.

The best thing about this recipe is that you can really make it yours. If you don't like onion, leave it out. If you don't have sweet potatoes, use canned pumpkin. Hate beets? Make orange sauce instead. Vary the herbs and spices you use to create different flavor combinations. Use more or less chicken broth for different textures.

It gets pretty thick once it's cooled down; thinning it out with some extra water or broth when you reheat is a good way to stretch it even further. This sauce freezes amazingly well. Using the bone broth recipe in this book instead of water will give you a wonderful depth of flavor, plus impart gut-healing benefits to the sauce.

After the Reintroduction Phase, if you discover that you can tolerate fermented foods and yeast, you can try adding a teaspoon of *umeboshi paste*, a salty, fermented plum puree that makes everything taste like … tomato … kind of. Well, as close as you'll get without adding an actual tomato.

1 onion, diced
2–4 garlic cloves, chopped
1 cup of chopped carrots
2 medium sweet potatoes, peeled and cubed (yields about 4 cups)
3 tablespoons pumpkin puree (optional for extra thick sauce)
3 tablespoons lemon juice
2 tablespoons balsamic or apple cider vinegar (use lemon juice
    if avoiding yeast)
Bone broth (page 204) or water, to cover
⅓ cup extra-virgin olive oil
1 cup water or bone broth, for thinning out sauce (optional)
Salt, to taste
Black pepper, to taste (optional)
8-ounce can of beets, pureed with juice
Choice of herbs: basil, oregano, and parsley*

*If using fresh herbs, use about ¼ to ½ cup each, depending on your tastes. If using dried, use 2 to 3 tablespoons of basil and parsley, and about 2 to 3 teaspoons of oregano. If you use Italian seasoning, make sure it doesn't contain tomato or red pepper!

1. In a large pot, sauté the onion and garlic in oil (ghee, coconut, olive, and/or avocado oil all work well) until they start to caramelize or brown.
2. Add the carrots, sweet potatoes, lemon juice, and vinegar and add enough bone broth or water to cover.
3. Bring to a boil, then lower the heat, cover with lid, and simmer for 20–30 minutes until the carrots and sweet potatoes are very soft. Add a little more water and the pumpkin puree if needed while cooking—you don't want the pot to dry out.
4. Add the olive oil and blend the contents of the pot until very smooth (in batches in a blender or with an immersion blender).
5. Return the sauce to the pot, and bring to a simmer over low heat. If the sauce becomes too thick too soon, add more water or bone broth to thin it out a bit. If it's too runny, simmer it for a while uncovered. The longer you cook it, the more concentrated the flavor.
6. Add salt and pepper to taste. By waiting until you've blended the sauce, you can tell how much it actually needs and you won't end up with something that is way too salty.
7. While your blended sauce is simmering, puree the contents of the can of beets (with the liquid included) in a blender until very smooth.
8. Add your herbs.
9. Add the beets to the pot, stir to combine and simmer for about 5 minutes. Be careful with this, if beets are cooked for too long they can turn brownish. We want our sauce to be red.
10. Add a little more water or chicken stock if needed, until the sauce is at the right consistency.

Original recipe adapted from glutenfreedairyfreenj.blogspot.ca

TOMATO-FREE KETCHUP
MAKES ABOUT 12 OUNCES

Yeast Alert! Make sure to wash the cranberries well and peel the apple. This recipe can be used for dipping, but also doubles as a pizza sauce. Just add lots of fresh herbs like basil and oregano and cut back a little on the allspice, cloves, and sweetener. If adding umeboshi paste, make sure to drastically cut back on the salt in this recipe.

   1 cup fresh cranberries
   1 large apple, peeled and cored
   2 medium carrots, peeled and chopped (1 cup)
   1 cup water
   1 tablespoon apple cider vinegar (use lemon juice if yeast intolerant)
   ⅛–¼ cup honey, maple syrup, or half coconut sugar and half stevia
   ½–1 teaspoon salt
   1 teaspoon onion powder
   ½ teaspoon allspice
   ⅛ teaspoon ground cloves

1. Combine all ingredients in a saucepan, cover with lid, and cook over medium low heat for 15 minutes, or until all ingredients are soft and mushy.
2. Blend with an immersion blender or in a food processor until smooth.
3. Chill and enjoy. Keeps in the fridge for one to two weeks. Can be frozen in batches and thaws beautifully.

Original recipe adapted from AmineRecipes.com.

HEALTH-BENT MOROCCAN CARROT SALAD
SERVES 4

1 pound carrots
3 tablespoons extra virgin olive oil
2 tablespoons fresh garlic, minced
1 tablespoon fresh mint, minced
2 tablespoons of unsweetened apple sauce
2 tablespoons white vinegar (lemon juice if yeast is an issue)
Salt to taste

1. Cut the tops and ends off of the carrots. Peel the carrots and discard the skins. Continue to peel the carrots until you've whittled them down as far as you can and place in a large bowl.
2. To a blender, add olive oil, garlic, mint, apple sauce, vinegar (or lemon juice), and mix until smooth.
3. Add mixture to carrots and toss to combine.

Recipe adapted from Primal Cravings: Your Favorite Foods Made Paleo, *by Brandon and Megan Keatley.*

CAULIFLOWER "RICE"
SERVES 4

The paleosphere is littered with various cauliflower rice recipes, all of which make great alternatives to rice. This basic recipe is limited only by your imagination. Serve it as the base to a stir-fry or dress it up by adding chopped onions or garlic or herbs to the pan when you heat your fat.

1 tablespoon ghee, tallow, lard, or coconut oil
1 head cauliflower, pulverized in food processor or hand grated
Salt and pepper to taste
Heat fat in sauté pan over low heat.
Add cauliflower and sauté for 5 minutes, stirring often.
Salt and pepper to taste

CHOPPED YELLOWFIN TUNA SALAD WITH AVOCADO AND BACON
MAKES 4 SERVINGS

This recipe comes courtesy of Mark Sisson, featured in his *Primal Blueprint Cookbook*. It's one of my favorites and so easy to make.

Oil for searing
1 pound yellowfin tuna steak
Salt and pepper to taste
¼ cup finely chopped red onion
1 avocado, peeled, pitted, and cut into small pieces
2 tablespoons finely chopped fresh dill or other herb
½ cup crumbled cooked bacon
2 tablespoons lemon juice

Heat heavy skillet over high heat 2 minutes. Brush tuna with oil and sprinkle lightly with salt and pepper. Place in the hot skillet and sear until browned on the outside, about 3 minutes per side for medium-rare, less for rare. Cool tuna; dice finely. Mix with other ingredients. Serve alone or over mixed greens.

HOW TO PREPARE ROOT VEGETABLES:
LET US COUNT THE WAYS
Sweet potatoes and yams

Thankfully, these delicious bundles of vitamins and nutrients are NOT nightshades. Prepare them as you would regular potatoes. If you don't like sweet potatoes, give them one more chance and try them prepared differently from how you normally eat them. Recently, I converted my father by making mashed sweet potatoes. He disliked baked sweet potatoes so much he didn't even want to try them. For some reason, when they were mashed with butter and salt, he couldn't get enough (just don't add a lot of milk, like you would with regular potatoes or you'll end up with soup). Sweet potatoes can be thrown in the microwave, just like regular potatoes, so they're a quick, easy dinner option. They're great deep-fried in tallow.

Taro root

You'll need to peel this one pretty aggressively—make sure you remove all the "hair" (and don't let it put you off!) and cut into desired shapes. Rinse and pat it dry after it's peeled. Cook it like potato; there is no need to boil first, unless you want boiled "potatoes." It's amazing deep-fried. I make tater tots for my kids out of taro and they love them. Use as a replacement for potatoes in casseroles, stews, soups, skillet dishes, etc.

Yuca root

Also known as cassava, manioc, or tapioca root. This one needs a little more prep, but it's worth it. Peel with a sharp paring knife. Cut into smallish pieces, depending on what you're going to do with it. Boil like potatoes for 30–40 minutes until it pierces easily with a fork. If you don't boil it enough, it will be mealy and white on the inside. You don't want to eat it like this, it may cause digestive upset if it's still raw. Once thoroughly cooked, remove from heat and drain. I like to fry the yuca root after it's boiled. You could also season it and bake until golden on a greased pan. **Note**: I don't recommend mashing yuca as an alternative to mashed potatoes. In this form, it tends to be too starchy and chewy.

Other Root Veggies

Most root vegetables are fairly versatile and can be easily found in your average supermarket. Our culture is just so focused on potato that we tend to forget about the other things.

Parsnips (look like yellow carrots) are something I grew up on. They are amazing fried or baked and have a sweet flavor. Panfry them in butter or roast them in the oven and you won't regret it.

Rutabaga and turnips have a strong flavor and may be an acquired taste. I've only ever had them boiled and mashed, but I'm sure there are tastier ways to prepare them. Michelle Tam at NomNomPaleo.com cubes them and roasts them with ghee, salt, and pepper. A delicious alternative to potato hash.

Kohlrabi (also known as German turnip and turnip cabbage) is an interesting vegetable. It can be eaten raw or cooked and tastes sort of like crunchy broccoli stems, with a slightly sweet flavor. Just peel, cut, and use your imagination.

Celeriac, or celery root, tastes just like celery but with a starchy, potato-like texture. It needs to be aggressively peeled, like yuca and taro. Add it to soups or stews in place of potatoes. Don't use too much of it in recipes like stew, unless you really like the flavor of celery.

There are so many root vegetables with which to experiment. Venture out of your comfort zone and try new ones. Sometimes the flavor can take some getting used to but over time, you'll come to love them as much as you once loved potatoes.

Building Your Personalized Recipe Collection

The following recipes are still Primal-paleo friendly, but they may contain one or two ingredients that you're going to need to test on yourself. Although these recipes may seem tempting, please wait until the Elimination Phase of your journey is complete before trying any of them.

TURMERIC EGG COFFEE
MAKES 1 SERVING

You'll remember that turmeric needs to be heated in order to be effective, and that it binds particularly well to the albumin in eggs. This recipe covers all the bases to make sure you receive turmeric's anti-inflammatory benefits.

1 cup hot black coffee or tea
¼ teaspoon turmeric
Generous pinch of salt
1 teaspoon sweetener: stevia, honey, or coconut sugar
Dash of cinnamon, cloves, cardamom, nutmeg, or other spices
   (optional)
2 eggs

1. Put all the ingredients, except the egg, into a blender. Turn blender on low.
2. Add the egg while the blender is still running.
3. Turn blender up to high, and watch the magic happen.
4. Pour your latte into your cup and enjoy hot.

SPICED CHAI LATTE
MAKES 1 SERVING

This versatile recipe is a master recipe of sorts. It calls for spiced ghee (I use Pure Indian Foods brand), but if you can't find it in your area, you can add 1 teaspoon to 1 tablespoon regular ghee with spices such as cardamom, cinnamon, ginger, cloves, or whatever you like. Chai, egg-nog, and pumpkin pie spice mixes work nicely. You'll want about ¼ to ½ teaspoon in total, but it will depend on your personal tastes. The flavor in the spiced ghee is very strong, so only use a little. (If you want to order some, check out the Resources section.)

   1 cup hot coffee or strong black tea
   1–2 tablespoons coconut oil, ghee, or coconut ghee
   1 teaspoon Pure Indian Foods Grass-Fed, Organic Digestive Ghee,
      or Indian Dessert Ghee
   Sweetener, to taste—Stevia, honey, maple syrup, or coconut sugar
   Pinch of salt
   1 egg or 2 egg yolks

1. Put all the ingredients, except the egg, into a blender. Turn blender on low.
2. Add the egg while the blender is still running.
3. Turn blender up to high until light-colored and frothy.
4. Pour your latte into your cup and enjoy hot.

REAL MAYONNAISE
MAKES APPROXIMATELY 1 CUP

I used to think you had to drizzle the oil in very slowly in order to make mayonnaise work, but my friend Orleatha taught me a secret that I'd like to share with you: how to make mayonnaise in under one minute. Get an immersion blender and a mason jar. That's all the equipment you need. If you don't own an immersion blender, place all the ingredients but the oil in a blender, and add oil one tablespoon at a time, very slowly.

1 large egg
1 tablespoon lemon juice
¼- ½ teaspoon salt
½ teaspoon ground mustard
Garlic, to taste (optional)
Herbs, to taste (optional)
1 cup avocado oil

1. Dump all the ingredients in the mason jar, in the order they appear.
2. Once all the ingredients are in the jar, stick the immersion blender in, and turn it on. Move it around and jiggle it a bit. You'll have mayonnaise in about 45 seconds. If for some reason you don't, and it just won't thicken, try adding an extra egg or a touch more lemon juice and reblend.
3. Store in the fridge. Keeps for about a week.

PREPARED MUSTARD
MAKES APPROXIMATELY 1 CUP

Making your own mustard means that you can skip the vinegar (if you need to) and use only ingredients that aren't triggers for you. Using lemon juice instead of vinegar will give the prepared mustard a bright, lively flavor, but if you can tolerate vinegar (or you want to test it) it is a more traditional choice. You can find mustard seeds in most grocery stores and Indian markets—the darker the seed, the stronger the taste. Mustard seeds can be problematic for some, so test this recipe out during the reintroduction phase.

⅓ cup mustard seeds
⅓ cup white wine vinegar, apple cider vinegar, or lemon juice
⅓ cup water (or white wine, if yeast and alcohol are not an issue)
1 tablespoon honey or maple syrup (optional)
1 teaspoon ground turmeric
¼-½ teaspoon salt
3 tablespoons warm water (if necessary)
Fresh grated horseradish root, to taste
  (optional; will give it a *major* kick)

1. Combine all ingredients, except for the horseradish and extra water, in a bowl. Cover and let stand for a couple days.
2. Put the mixture in a blender and pulse until it's as smooth as possible. Add the extra water if the mustard is too thick.
3. Add the horseradish, if using, and blend.

Note: The prepared mustard will keep up to six months in the fridge, but it's best used within one month.
Original recipe adapted from www.davidlebovitz.com

TARRAGON CREAM FISH SAUCE
MAKES APPROXIMATELY 1 CUP

This sauce goes really well with fish—especially white fish. Using home-made mayonnaise will give you a thicker end result, as the real egg in your mayo will cook in the oven while the fish is baking. I also like to use this sauce as a fish and chicken marinade. I pour the extra marinade on the fish while it's baking.

½ cup mayonnaise (page 217)
1 tablespoon prepared mustard (page 218)
¼ cup lime juice
2 teaspoons dried tarragon (2 tablespoons if using fresh)
Salt to taste
Black pepper to taste (optional)

Combine all ingredients in a small bowl and whisk to combine. Add extra lime juice if the mixture is too thick, or more mayonnaise if it's too thin. Pour over fish and bake, or use as a dipping sauce.

NUT BUTTERS & NUT MILK

If you tolerate nuts then you have an amazing variety of nut butters available to you, without all the sugar and the hydrogenated oils that normally accompany store-bought peanut butter. Almond butter, cashew butter, or macadamia nut butter are available in many health stores, but you can easily make your own for a lot less money.

If you have a Vitamix or other high-powered blender, you can make your own nut butter in a matter of minutes. Just throw the nuts in and turn it on. That's all there is to it—just like the coconut cream recipe. Or you can add some filtered water to the nut butter, and turn it back on. Now, you have cashew milk. Or almond milk. Or whatever-nut-you-had-in-the-blender milk. If you would like to make a big batch of nut milk, a good rule of thumb is one cup of nuts to four cups of filtered water, or follow the Coconut Milk recipe on page 205.

BANANA CRÈPES

MAKES 2 SERVINGS

1 banana, mashed
2 eggs
½ teaspoon gluten-free, alcohol-free vanilla (optional)
Cinnamon, nutmeg, or whatever spices you like (optional)
Salt to taste (optional)

1. Combine all ingredients in a small bowl or a food processor until smooth.
2. Heat a griddle or frying pan to medium-low heat. (Non-stick works best for this.)
3. Add butter or coconut oil to the pan.
4. Pour ⅛ to ¼ cup of batter into the frying pan and spread to desired size. Cook approximately 1 to 2 minutes per side, or until golden brown.
5. Add cut up fruit, nuts, or whatever Primal-friendly ingredient you like to the crèpes, roll up, and enjoy.

BANANA-COCONUT PANCAKES

Follow the recipe for Banana Crèpes and add ½–¾ cup of unsweetened shredded coconut. The pancakes are thicker than the crèpes and will stay together well.

KOMBUCHA

Kombucha is fizzy and refreshing, just like soda. Since it is a fermented food, so you'll be getting lots of B vitamins, vitamin K, and beneficial bacteria and yeast instead of high fructose corn syrup.

In order to make this fermented sweet tea beverage, you need to get your hands on a kombucha SCOBY—a symbiotic culture of bacteria and yeast—that is sometimes called a mushroom. If you can't find a SCOBY locally, you can order one on the Internet. You can also find detailed instructions online, including YouTube videos, to get you started.

Although kombucha is very nutritious, if you've discovered that yeast is a trigger for you, it's best to skip this one.

GRAIN-FREE TORTILLAS
MAKES ABOUT EIGHT 4-INCH TORTILLAS

Don't roll them out too thin or they'll break apart! This is a good recipe to try to see if you can tolerate coconut flour; while it doesn't cause leaky gut directly, coconut flour can cause gas and bloating in some people. Best to find out early if that's you.

1 cup tapioca flour
¼ cup coconut flour
¼ teaspoon aluminum-free baking soda
½ teaspoon cream of tartar
¼ cup lard or palm oil
¼–½ teaspoon salt
½ cup boiling water

1. Sift all dry ingredients. Add lard or shortening to dry ingredients, mixing with a fork to form crumbles.
2. Add hot water into dry ingredients mixing until dough-like. (Don't be afraid to use your hands!)
3. Form 2-inch balls, place between two sheets of parchment or wax paper and press into flat discs.
4. Place in ungreased skillet until top begins to dry around the edges—the underside will be slightly brown.
5. Remove from pan and let cool before eating. They will become more pliable as they cool.

Recipe courtesy of Orleatha Smith. This recipe can be found at www.lvlhealth.com.

SAUERKRAUT
MAKES 1 QUART

Raw sauerkraut is amazingly easy to make and delivers beneficial bacteria in every bite. Although you may not like the taste of it on its own at first, it pairs very well with any type of meat. Trust me—you will develop a taste for it after a while, especially when you see what it can do for your health.

Raw sauerkraut is available in some grocery stores in the refrigerated section but it is incredibly expensive. Making it at home takes minutes and costs about a buck.

1 head of cabbage, shredded.
4 tablespoons Redmond's Real Salt (or other high-quality sea salt)

1. Shred the cabbage in a food processor, or chop it up any way you like. Smaller pieces work best.
2. In a large bowl, sprinkle the salt on the cabbage and massage it with your hands until lots of water starts coming out of the cabbage. I know it seems like a lot of salt, but it's necessary for the fermentation process.
3. Pack the cabbage and juice into a clean mason jar. Pack it down well until the juice covers the top of the cabbage.
4. Seal the jar and store in a cool, dry place for approximately 4 days, or until you like the taste. Mix, taste, and pack it down again each day. You can let it ferment for as long as you like; the longer it ferments, the more sour and the less salty it will be. When it is sour enough for you, you can store it in the fridge and it will stop fermenting.
5. Save the leftover juice to add to your next batch, as it makes an excellent starter. You can also use it to ferment other vegetables.
6. Try the basic recipe first, then venture out and add other vegetables and fruits to the cabbage. Carrots and apples work well.
7. The color of the cabbage and any other vegetables you use will change and get darker. This is normal.
8. If the sauerkraut has mold on the top or smells really bad (other than the way sauerkraut usually smells), then toss it and start over.

You may have introduced some bad bacteria by mistake and you don't want to eat it and get sick.

9. Spices such as caraway, anise, fennel, and celery seed are wonderful additions. Each will give a completely different flavor to the finished product.

10. Adding sauce to the sauerkraut when it's done is a great way to get kids to eat it. I like to mix cabbage, carrots, apples, a teaspoon of celery seed, and add a sauce when it's finished fermenting.

HONEY GINGER SESAME SAUCE
MAKES 2/3 CUP

This tastes great poured over the sauerkraut dish. Add some lemon juice and you can also use it as a salad dressing, or a marinade for chicken.

2 tablespoons coconut oil, melted
2 tablespoons olive oil
2 tablespoons sesame oil
2–4 tablespoons raw honey
½ tablespoons fresh grated ginger

Mix all ingredients together and add to sauerkraut. Mix well and serve at room temperature.

FAUX-COCCIA BREAD
MAKES 2 MEDIUM-LARGE FLATBREADS

This flatbread is amazing on its own and can even be used for pizza crust! Rolling it thinner will result in more even baking and a slightly crispier texture. You'll notice this recipe has flax and eggs in it. Tapioca can also be problematic for some. Try it and see how you react to the ingredients.

3 cups tapioca flour
1 cup coconut flour
½ cup golden flax meal
½ teaspoon oregano
½ teaspoon granulated garlic
½ teaspoon rosemary
1 teaspoon salt
½ teaspoon baking soda
1 teaspoon cream of tartar
1 ¼ cups water
⅓ cup olive oil
2 eggs beaten
½ cup coconut milk

1. Preheat oven to 400 degrees.
2. Sift dry ingredients in a medium sized bowl.
3. Whisk in the wet ingredients. Let the dough sit for a minute or two; it will thicken up.
4. Form two balls. Place one ball between a piece of parchment paper (bottom) and a piece of wax paper (top) then roll to desired thickness.
5. Place on pizza pan or cookie sheet (with parchment paper) and bake for 20 minutes, or until brown.

Recipe courtesy of Orleatha Smith. This recipe can be found at www.lvlhealth.com.

LEMON-LIME GUMMY SQUARES
MAKES 4-6 SERVINGS

This recipe is quick to make and is perfect for cravings for sour candy. You'll be getting the benefits of grass-fed gelatin, as well as vitamins and antioxidants from the fruit you use—but none of the artificial garbage that's in commercial candy. Gelatin is great for your skin, hair, and nails. To make this fun for kids, pour the mixture into fun silicone molds, or use small cookie cutters after it's set. If you're using a pan, make sure it's glass or ceramic. **Note:** Stick to the lemon-lime version of these gummies if you're avoiding yeast and make sure to limit the amount of sweetener you use.

⅔ cup lemon juice
⅓ cup lime juice
¼ cup water (optional; it will be very sour without it)
1-2 tablespoons honey or maple syrup
5 tablespoons Great Lakes grass-fed gelatin (orange or red container)
Zest from lemons or limes, optional

1. In a pot over medium-low heat, whisk the juice, water, and honey or maple syrup together. Taste for sweet-sour balance; add more sweetener or water if desired.
2. Measure out the gelatin into a separate bowl. While still whisking the juice mixture, slowly sprinkle the gelatin into the mixture. Keep whisking to avoid lumps. Continue until all the gelatin has been incorporated into the mixture.
3. Remove from heat and add optional zest. Stir to combine.
4. Pour the mixture into silicone molds, or a glass or ceramic dish. The smaller the pan, the thicker the gummies will be. Chill in the fridge to set, approximately 30-60 minutes.

Variations: You can add fruit to make different colored and flavored gummy squares! Just take away the water in the above recipe, replace with one cup of blended fruit (any kind, except for pineapple), and increase the gelatin to 6 tablespoons. You may not need any extra sweetener if you use fruit—taste before you add any!
Original recipe adapted from www.balancedbites.com

BLUEBERRY LEMON CHEESECAKE
MAKES 8 SERVINGS

This is another amazing recipe from *The Autoimmune Paleo Cookbook* by Mickey Trescott. Save this one for special occasions—no matter how good the ingredients are for you, cheesecake is not an everyday food. Well, OK, just make it this once to test it, you need to make sure it's good enough for company.

Time: 1 hour, plus 12 hours to set

For the Crust
3 cups dates, pitted and soaked for 5 minutes in warm water
1 cup coconut oil, melted
⅓ cup coconut flour
⅓ cup shredded coconut
⅛ teaspoon salt

For the Filling
1 cup raw honey, softened
1 cup coconut cream, softened (page 206)
¾ cup coconut oil, softened
3 cups frozen blueberries
4 tablespoons tapioca starch
1 teaspoon vanilla extract (alcohol & gluten free)
1 lemon, juiced and zested
⅛ teaspoon salt

Fresh blueberries for garnish

1. Place the jars of coconut oil, coconut cream, and raw honey in a pan with very hot water to soften.
2. To prepare the crust, preheat your oven to 325 degrees. Strain the dates and place in a food processor or high-powered blender with the melted coconut oil. Blend for 30 seconds or so until a chunky paste forms. Be warned that you may have to stop and scrape the sides if you are using a blender, and the oil may not completely mix

with the dates, but the crust will still turn out fine. Combine the coconut flour, shredded coconut, and salt in a bowl. Add the date paste and mix thoroughly. Place the mixture into the bottom of a pie dish, using your fingers to push it up and form it around the sides evenly. Bake for 30-35 minutes, until the crust browns and hardens a little. The texture will still be soft until it finishes cooling. Set aside while you make the filling.

3. To make the filling, combine the raw honey, coconut butter, coconut oil, and frozen blueberries in a saucepan on low heat. Stir until the berries are no longer frozen and the mixture is warm, about 5 minutes. Transfer to a blender and add the tapioca starch, vanilla extract, lemon juice, zest, and salt. Blend on high for about a minute, until completely mixed. Pour carefully onto the crust.

4. Set in the refrigerator undisturbed for at least 12 hours to allow the cake to cool and completely harden.

5. When it is solid, decorate the top of the cake with fresh blueberries.

Note: Keeps in a cool place unrefrigerated, but safest to keep in the refrigerator. Leftover slices can be frozen for later.

Reprinted with permission by Mickey Trescott, The Autoimmune Paleo Cookbook, *2013.*

CHOCOLATE CHIP COOKIES
MAKES 12-14 COOKIES

Some people choose to leave eggs and nuts in their diet during the elimination phase, or can't wait to reintroduce them. If this is you, then this recipe is perfect. Leaving the chocolate chips out altogether is recommended for beginners or for those who are still actively flaring up. You can substitute slivered almonds for the chocolate instead. When I use chocolate chips, I use Real Life brand; they contain no dairy or soy, and can be found at progressive supermarkets.

1 cup almond butter
1 egg
Honey to taste (around 1 teaspoon to 2 tablespoons)
1 teaspoon gluten-free, alcohol-free vanilla
½ teaspoon aluminum-free baking soda
¼–½ teaspoon salt
⅛–¼ cup chocolate chips (optional)

1. Preheat oven to 350 degrees and line a cookie sheet with parchment paper.
2. Mix all ingredients together in a bowl, folding in the chocolate chips last.
3. Drop about 1 tablespoon of the batter onto the prepared cookie sheet, keeping cookies about 2 inches apart.
4. Bake at 350 degrees for 9 to 10 minutes. Cookies will still be soft and will need to "set" (rest) for approximately 10 minutes before you remove them from the pan.
5. Once the cookies have rested, remove them from the pan and allow to cool on a wire rack or eat them immediately. If there are any left, seal in plastic bags or a glass container. They will be extra chewy if you store them in the fridge.

BEANS

As hard as I've tried, I can't find substitutions for beans; there's nothing quite like their texture and taste out there, except for ... beans. Your best bet is just to avoid dishes that contain them. You can also try soaking dry beans for 24-48 hours (rinsing often) before thoroughly cooking them to see if disabling some of the antinutrients allows you to eat them. Research traditional ways of soaking, sprouting, and fermenting legumes before you do this, so you can make sure you're doing it right.

DIY LARD & TALLOW

This process is very simple to do yourself at home. Ask your butcher for fat scraps. They will more than likely give them to you for free. Bring them home, remove any muscle meat, and cut them into 1-inch cubes. Freezing them for about thirty minutes before you do this can help make it easier.

Put the fat cubes into an ovenproof pot or pan, and put them in the oven uncovered at approximately 250 degrees Fahrenheit for a few hours. Check on them every so often and give them a stir if you feel the need. Once it seems like there's no more fat left to come out of the cracklings (which will be left over), take it out of the oven and let it cool a bit. You can then strain the fat through cheesecloth or a clean, cotton dishtowel into mason jars. Store it in the fridge or the freezer, where it will keep for months.

For more recipes, autoimmune-friendly cookbooks, and to find out where to purchase specific ingredients mentioned in this chapter, please refer to *Resources*.

Staples to Keep on Hand

- Grass-fed ground beef, cuts of meat, and poultry
- Canned tuna, sardines, mackerel
- Nitrate-free bacon
- Bone broth (page 204)
- Avocado
- Canned pumpkin
- Green plantains
- Sweet potatoes, yams, and other root vegetables such as beets or parsnips
- Your favorite fresh (or frozen) organic fruits and vegetables
- Tapioca flour (for reintroduction phase)
- Oils: coconut oil, avocado oil
- Animal fat: ghee, tallow, lard, duck fat
- Sweeteners: liquid stevia, raw honey, maple syrup, and/or coconut sugar
- Sea salt, Himalayan pink salt, or Redmond's-brand Real Salt
- Fresh herbs
- Onions, garlic
- Coconut cream
- Unsweetened, shredded coconut
- Coconut milk (page 205)

CHAPTER ELEVEN
Frequently Asked Questions

have been on the autoimmune paleo diet for a week, taking a million supplements, apple cider vinegar shots, no caffeine, no smoking, no nightshades, etc., and today I woke up with a boil the size of a quarter. I've actually had it all summer long, but it never came to a head and there have been times when I thought it might even go away. Now it's worse than ever. What am I doing wrong?

I know the feeling. The old "Whadd'ya mean, I haven't lost a single pound?!? I've been on this crappy diet an entire WEEK!" kind of feeling. The way you feel when you are so desperate for something to work that you get fatalistic if it doesn't happen overnight. But think about it: if you have had a boil for several months, and it's been bothering you greatly during all that time, how can you possibly expect your body to fully drain it, heal it, and prevent others from flaring up within a matter of days? Your body is in the middle of an inflammatory process and it is going to take way longer for all that to calm down. Plus, you are dealing with insulin sensitivity, leaky gut, and the out-of-balance hormones. It takes time to reverse all that.

Other things to consider are all those new supplements you are taking. Apple cider vinegar, for instance, should be eliminated during the elimination phase of the autoimmune paleo diet. (See chapter eight: *Phase I: Elimination Diet*.) Also, make sure your supplements are labeled "yeast free," especially if you are taking vitamin B. Other possible triggers include medication, birth control pills, and, if you are eating any kind of packaged food, be sure to check the label for hidden ingredients that cause gut irritation. And finally, evaluate your stress levels. Are you trying to do too much at once, causing your body to send signals to your gut and making it inflamed? Some people experience an attack of their autoimmune issues when they first try something new. Sometimes things get a little worse before they get better. Calm down, take it easy, and cut yourself some slack.

Even after your triggers have been addressed, it can take months for your gut to heal. For some of us, it will never heal completely. That's right—the longer a person suffers from HS, the less likely that person will recover and go into full remission. If your intestinal damage is extensive, you may fight a battle for many years to come. However, you'll find the cleaner you eat and the cleaner you live your life, the better and better you will continue to feel. Your HS symptoms will become less painful and less frequent as a result. I suffered for over twenty years and was able to get rid of it, but it took me about three years before I went into complete remission, so please be patient with yourself and the process. And whatever you do, don't give up after a week. Give it at least thirty to sixty days and you should see some significant improvement in at least some area of you life.

I started the autoimmune protocol (AIP) thirteen days ago and have not cheated at all. I have a really bad flare-up under both my arms that were there before I started the diet. They got a little better, but now they are worse again. My question is should I start to look at other things to cut out of the diet, such as fruit? Or should I wait a little longer before cutting anything else out?

Things sometimes get worse before they get better. People often report a worsening of symptoms, especially pain and inflammation, when the healing process begins. These reactions should subside after a few weeks but if they don't, then it's your first clue that something is still out of whack. If you are not cheating on the diet, then you may want to look into external sources of stress and inflammation, such as omega-6 intake (see page 88), inadequate sleep (page 134), or too much fructose (page 106). Gentle exercise can also work wonders to reduce inflammation and normalize insulin levels.

Please remember that it takes time to heal from this condition. You may even flare up again in a few months and have difficulty pinpointing the cause. This doesn't mean that what you're doing isn't working. Compare your current condition to the way your HS used to be. If it's worse now, then change what you're doing. If it's better, then you're on the right path. However, wait for a couple months before you bail on what you're doing now.

Tissue damage can linger long after an autoimmune attack subsides. The body can heal itself, but only if the autoimmune attack is stopped from further ravaging bodily tissues. Working together with a naturopath or functional diagnostic nutrition expert would probably be a good idea if you've been at it for several months and haven't seen a lessening of symptoms.

If you already had the flare-ups under your arms before you started the AIP, don't worry too much—they can take quite a while to subside and heal. If you have new ones appearing, it would be a matter of concern. Now, that being said, I have personally found that once I healed my gut, if I introduced a trigger food I would break out but it would be small, not painful, and would go away within a day or two. If you have inflammation that is worsening over time, I would definitely take a closer look at what you're putting in your mouth or talk to a doctor.

Any tips on how to start a paleo diet without wanting to kill yourself for a donut?

The first few weeks can be hard, but once your body adapts and starts burning fat instead of sugar (approximately twenty-one days), the cravings should subside and it will be easier to handle.

I encourage you to explore the Primal and paleo lifestyles more fully. Look into books like *The Primal Blueprint*, by Mark Sisson, or *The Paleo Solution* by Robb Wolf. Go online and find a support network of people who are living the same lifestyle as you. You can start with the forum on PrimalGirl.com.

I also find that being "stubborn" about certain ingredients (for me it's wheat and potato) is helpful; I will under no circumstances eat anything that has wheat or potatoes in it, but I may indulge if it's made with tapioca flour or rice. This is where knowing your triggers and how much you can get away with without penalty is helpful. For instance, I can enjoy a little sugar on one day, but if I consume a little bit of sugar for four consecutive days, I will pay the price with a boil.

Which brings me to vilifying the food you're trying to avoid. When you have a direct negative reaction to something, it makes it less appetizing. I have a personal vendetta against things with potato in them; they make me sick, inflamed, and bring me pain. I associate potatoes with illness. This makes it much easier to say no to a handful of chips in a moment of weakness.

I also have Hashimoto's Thyroiditis,* and I've read that it's sometimes associated with HS. How do I get rid of both of them? How are they connected?

* You can substitute PCOS, diabetes, arthritis, eczema, or myriad autoimmune conditions out there for the Hashimoto's.

I've received many questions from people who suffer from more than one autoimmune issue at a time. Guess what? It's all part of the same problem: autoimmunity.

Your body is being attacked on more than one front. When autoimmunity decides to strike multiple systems in your body—such as the joints, skin, kidneys, blood cells, heart, and lungs—all at once, you end up with what the doctors call lupus. When it attacks your pancreas, you get diabetes. When it attacks your hair follicles, you get HS. The good news is that once you heal your leaky gut and stay away from your triggers, you should see relief from all other autoimmune conditions. If you don't, seek out a naturopath or a doctor who specializes in autoimmune issues. For more information on this, check out chapter three, *Autoimmunity 101.*

My doctor says that making changes to my diet won't do anything and that I have to go on antibiotics or have surgery. What do you say to that?

Honestly? I would ask that doctor which recent medical study he is using to reach that conclusion. I would then hand him a copy of this book, have him read it, and ask him that question again. But then again, I don't always make the right decisions in doctor's offices, and I've pissed many of them off.

This is a hard one. So many of us have been "fobbed off" by the medical community for so many years that we don't even bother going to the doctors anymore. There are those of us who still have some faith, but it's hard to stay loyal to a fatalistic doctor who doesn't know how to fix you and only prescribes treatments that other people have already proven don't work.

If you've read the stories and information in this book, you will have everything you need to make a decision for yourself. Because YOU are the one who is going to have to heal from surgery. Only YOU can decide if it is right for you in the first place. YOU are the one that is going to have to deal with the side effects of the drugs and pay for the prescriptions. Only YOU can decide if that is what you want to do.

Doctors are there to advise us of the different courses of treatments, not to tell us what to do or make us feel guilty. That is not their job.

A problem I'm having with "going paleo" is the higher fat content. I, like most dieters, believed the hype that I should eat LESS fat ... and that was working for me because I have no gallbladder. I'm hoping that eating sauerkraut and taking digestive enzymes will help me with that issue. Any tips?

We have been brainwashed, people. Fat is not bad for us. In fact, when I started eating more *real* fat, many of my health problems completely went away. My cholesterol went down. As did my weight and systemic inflammation. My hair and skin looked awesome. My brain function, mood, and energy levels also stabilized. Increasing my fat intake was the best thing I'd ever done.

I don't have any problem digesting fat whatsoever—my problem is digesting carbohydrates—so this was a tough question for me to answer.

Luckily, Orleatha Smith, a certified holistic lifestyle coach and nutritionist, is in the same boat as you. She underwent gastric bypass surgery several years ago, before she found the Paleo lifestyle, and also had her gallbladder removed.

At the time, Orleatha was told that a lowfat diet was the way to go and that she wouldn't be able to digest fat for the rest of her life. One of the reasons I love her so much is because she doesn't just accept news that she doesn't like; she does research, experiments on herself, and finds a solution that works. I'll let her answer your question:

> Unrefined coconut oil is made up of short and medium chain fatty acids. It does not need pancreatic enzymes or bile salts for digestion like other kinds of fats—even the good fats like animal fats. Using coconut oil also allows you to break down and absorb more of the fat-soluble vitamins that you need, like A, D, E and K. Since it is anti-viral and anti-bacterial it may increase detoxifying, healing reactions and symptoms so it is important to start introducing coconut oil slowly then gradually increase it.

Orleatha is now able to digest all types of fat. Just keep in mind that this took a while to accomplish; she didn't go from surgery to inhaling a 16-ounce steak in one sitting overnight. Ask Orleatha more questions about eating fat and gastric bypass at LVLHealth.com.

I recently cut chicken out of my diet because I suspected it was my trigger. I cut it out two weeks before Thanksgiving. At the beginning of December, I was craving chicken pasta so I ate some. Within TWO hours my bumps were swollen and pissed off. So I waited four weeks and tried again, and again it happened. So I bought some organic chicken and cooked it, NOTHING happened. Today, my daughter wanted chicken nuggets so I made them from Food Lion, and I took TWO bites. In less than an hour my worst bump is aching and burning. I wanted to share this in case you had any suggestions or ideas on whether this might be a true trigger or if it is just a coincidence. By the way, I had hardly any flare-ups during the "cut out" period.

When your gut is leaky, it allows proteins from everything you're eating into your bloodstream. It may very well be that your body has developed a sensitivity to the proteins in chicken, although my initial instinct would be to look elsewhere.

There are a couple red flags in your email. First off, you mention that you were craving "chicken pasta." Pasta is wheat. It can also be made with potato, soy, corn, quinoa and tons of other gut irritants. What was in the pasta sauce? Tomato? Peppers? Soy? Dairy?

Chicken nuggets are loaded with things that cause leaky gut and reactions in HS sufferers: wheat, corn, dairy, soy, nightshades, sugar, high fructose corn syrup, chemicals, stabilizers, etc. Don't jump to the conclusion that the chicken is the problem when you have a million other things on your plate.

When you ate the organic chicken, what did you eat it with? If you ate it by itself and didn't react, then I believe you have your answer.

You may also be experiencing low stomach acid, which can cause difficulties digesting protein and cause leaky gut. For more information on low stomach acid, check out ChrisKresser.com.

I have HS and it's starting to get worse. The doctors have tried all sorts of antibiotics, and, as it turns out, I'm allergic to them and break out in hives when I take just about anything. They aren't willing to talk about any other treatments. I've been doing research on my own and have come across your site and it's given me a lot of hope. I would really like to heal myself through food.

Keeping a diary isn't a problem; that's the easy part. It's the food that's the issue. I don't like to eat meat and there are certain types I flat out refuse to eat (it's a compassion thing on my part). So what's a girl to do? Live with HS or eat a diet that emotionally wrecks me? Or is there some sort of happy medium where I could eat meat sometimes and stick to fruit and vegetables the rest of the time?

This is another tough one. I certainly can't get into the whole vegan-vegetarian debate. For more information on that, I suggest reading Lierre Keith's *The Vegetarian Myth*. However, something I can tell you about the Primal-paleo community is that we're actually just like vegetarians in a lot of regards: we hate concentrated animal feeding operations (CAFOs), animal cruelty, and senseless slaughter. We believe that the animals we eat should be raised humanely, treated with dignity, have access to space and sunshine, and eat a diet specific to their species.

There is proof that animals raised this way are better for us—grass-fed beef is actually a good source of omega-3 fatty acids, for example, whereas corn-fed beef is high in omega-6 fatty acids, which can cause inflammation in the body if it's the predominate fatty acid in the diet. Like humans, animals that don't eat a species-specific diet—that is, the foods they evolved on and their bodies are designed for—get very sick and need medication like antibiotics. There's a lot of talk about food quality in the paleo community, and eating organic, pasture-raised animals tops our list of priorities.

If you aren't eating meat for religious or compassionate reasons, then choosing quality over quantity and buying directly from farmers who treat their animals well may help you feel better about your decision.

That said, there's nothing that says you need to eat a lot of meat on this diet. As long as you are avoiding your trigger foods, healing your gut, and fueling your body properly with whole foods, you should see improvement in your HS. I do know someone who put his HS into complete remission by eating a strict raw vegan diet. He swears he's in remission because he cut out meat. I don't have the heart to tell him that his strict diet cuts out *all* the major trigger foods, including wheat, legumes, dairy, and potatoes. Had he chosen a vegetarian diet instead of raw vegan one without all the dairy and grains, he would have had a much different outcome.

Our diets end up being as individual as we are. I know someone who is quite prominent in the primal community who doesn't eat red meat at all—she eats eggs and fish instead—because she just doesn't like how she feels when she eats meat. You may be this way. If you're avoiding meat simply for ethical reasons, please consider buying directly from a small farm, ordering meat from progressive farmers online, or asking your butcher if he can stock humanely raised, grass-fed meats for you.

Got a question of your own? Feel free to post it on PrimalGirl.com! Opening up and sharing your story helps others deal with their situation.

CHAPTER TWELVE

Success Stories

My original blog posts about the connection between HS and diet have been up for almost two years now and I still continue to get hundreds of hits each day. As people connect their HS with what they are eating, the success stories are rolling in.

I've included a few of these stories here, in the hope that anyone who is still on the fence about moving forward with a paleo autoimmune diet will be convinced, and also to give support and hope to those who are just starting on their path to healing.

Thank you to everyone who has submitted success stories. By sharing what works for you, we can help other people find what works for them.

We'll kick off the testimonials with Wendy's story, a tale of a dynamic young woman who took matters into her own hands to end her suffering with HS. Much like myself, Wendy didn't have a lot of luck with doctors or conventional treatment, so she took the natural route and healed herself using Primal/paleo foods. Wendy's story is inspiring and closely mirrors my own—right down to the person who introduced her to this lifestyle: her brother. She has also contributed information in chapter six, *Wound Care* (page 111), about how she took care of her flare-ups. Since her boils were in a very delicate area, she provides invaluable insight to those of you suffering the same fate.

I've suffered from HS for over seventeen years. It's located exclusively in the labial tissues, although early on I had a massive boil form at just under the bikini line, on the groin. The labial boils never get larger than a large pea—but the pain of those "peas" (often multiples at a time) has often been unbearable. I missed a lot of time at work and socializing with friends and family as a result of HS. Sitting and walking during flares were invariably excruciating. Laying down with legs spread to relieve pressure on the labia and in order to avoid rubbing motions from walking was one of the only reliable ways to get some relief, though the itching and pain was never totally gone.

When the boils first showed up in my mid-twenties, I worried they were herpes. I was tested for every STD on the planet and when results were negative, I insisted on getting retested several times in repetition. Nothing, not even herpes type 1 (mouth cold sores), which can occur on the genitals. I had several biopsies taken during flare-ups. The only result from the biopsies was "generalized inflammation."

I began seeing a "pelvic floor specialist" gyno who was part of a sub-specialty practice at a prestigious university hospital. At first she thought lichens planus, then said no. She then arrived finally at HS, an autoimmune disease. I'd never heard of it before. She prescribed antibiotics, steroid shots in the hoo-ha (to "reduce inflammation"—those were fun) and proposed surgery as an option if things "got much worse." I did the antibiotics, kept the area clean regularly, and underwent several rounds of the shots. Surgery was too scary for me. Once those delicate labial tissues are altered or removed, it's permanent. Eventually I basically "gave up" and stopped seeing her or seeking medical "treatment." I resigned myself to the flare-ups and tried to manage them as best I could on my own.

Before I stopped seeing the specialist, her last "treatment" was homeopathic, which I much later understood to be a total joke. Even better, it was a belladonna "remedy." Talk about ironic. Luckily, I had to travel out of my way to a special compounding pharmacy to even get it, so I didn't waste too much money on it in the end. The last thing the specialist told me was that giving up caffeine would probably help. It about killed me, but I did it: I gave up my beloved coffee.

Fast forward over a decade to early October 2011: I was obese and knew I needed to lose weight. I'd managed to starve/exercise myself down about thirty pounds, but couldn't tolerate the lifestyle longer than about six months. My brother then told me about something he was trying called the "paleo/primal diet" and his surprising, excellent results. I decided that however hard it would be for me to give up things like wheat, grains, sugar, and processed "food," I had to try it due to how well my brother was doing with weight loss.

I was extremely strict about it for the first thirty days. I quit wheat, all other grains, and grain products cold turkey. I didn't eat "safe" starches like potatoes because I believed I was already in the early stages of insulin resistance, and was serious about losing weight. So avoiding starchy stuff, sugars, and grains were the initial priority.

I felt amazing after the first month and lost almost ten pounds, so I kept going. I never kept super strict paleo, other than to nearly perfectly not eat wheat, sugar, sweeteners, or most grains (very occasional rice—like once a quarter, if that, with sushi). I continued to lose weight without having to work at it, other than prepare primal meals at home.

After a few months had passed, I suddenly realized I hadn't had my "normal" once or twice a month HS flare. Typically, walking and sitting during flares had been such an utter nightmare that coping with that sort of pain had become a regular part of every month. The flares also normally clustered around my periods—which are very regular (no PCOS here, luckily) —so I always knew when to expect the misery to begin.

I'd stopped taking antibiotics many years ago. I'd stopped doing anything except just trying to keep things clean, sometimes self-lancing when things got too agonizing in order to drain the pus and blood, and generally trying to keep a stiff upper lip. My dear, understanding husband had long understood since HS first appeared that because of its location, I quickly lost interest in certain oral intimacies that many married couples take for granted. I felt so gross and very broken "down there."

So, when I noticed a solid three to four months of eating Primally had passed without a single HS flare, I sat straight up—without pain!—and began a food diary which I kept for the rest of 2012. I continued with it and ate wheat exactly three times: on our anniversary, for my birthday, and on Thanksgiving. Each "wheat cheat" also involved the usual sugar (dessert items). Flare-ups came right on the heels of each cheat. So I no longer care if it's wheat, some other grain, or sugar—I avoid all grains and sugar like the plague. Such motivations to avoid both have made the lifestyle incredibly easy for me.

I've even started drinking real coffee again, cautiously at first, but for the past seven-plus months I have been drinking two giant mugs of dark roast (about 32 ounces) every single morning with no problems whatsoever. I'm amazed that I gave up something I enjoyed so much for nearly a decade. For nothing, as it turns out.

So, in short: I don't eat any type of grains or grain products. I'm still really good at avoiding seed oils—I make my own olive oil mayo and all salad dressings/sauces. I cook with coconut oil and butter. I eat as much clean saturated fat as I can stuff myself with along with animal protein (as much grass-fed as I can afford), and vegetables—mostly of the leafy green or simply green variety: greens, asparagus, brussel sprouts, broccoli, cabbage, etc.

After reintroducing potatoes at about the six-month mark, I have found that I appear to be OK with them in moderation (once a week), as well as cooked tomatoes, and the occasional eggplant dish.

None appear to have any association with HS flares. I have been eating a lot of eggs from the beginning, and they also appear to be fine for me. I no longer buy or eat processed food of any kind, and my sweet tooth has pretty much become extinct. I can tolerate small amounts of dairy—heavy cream in my coffee, a few bits of stinky cheese and buttermilk. Those are my "cheats"—and they appear to be fine for me as well.

Ever since late 2011—for the first time in over seventeen years—I have been in complete remission from HS except for the three flares I documented after eating wheat and sugar.

What drives me crazy is the bizarre idea in mainstream medicine that what we take into our bodies—what we eat—has little or no bearing on autoimmune disease. All it took was for me to become my own guinea pig to make it crystal clear that there's an undeniable connection.

I've since read Robb Wolf, Mark Sisson, Gary Taubes and Loren Cordain. I give thanks every day that my brother clued me in to Primal/paleo eating, and I've learned so much. My husband has also benefited—he was obese, like me, and is now within 10 lbs of his goal weight. Not to give TMI, but the improvement in a certain part of our intimate life together has been like a miracle. Tears of gratitude have been shed.

When I look back at all the years I suffered so needlessly, it makes me angry. Then I remember how easy it is for me to stay in remission. And I feel joyful all over again. I have my life back, and I'm still young!

So, PrimalGirl, thank you again for helping to spread the word about HS and the autoimmune connection to what we eat. I am utterly convinced that in one way or another, those of us who suffer from HS have most certainly triggered an autoimmune response via an offending ingested substance, whether it's wheat, another grain, soy, legumes, nightshades, sugar, or something else.

Following an autoimmune protocol diet and keeping a strict food diary are the first vital steps that anyone suffering from HS can take toward freeing themselves from so much of the suffering this horrific disease causes."

—Wendy

I've been strictly paleo since the beginning of August 2012, and auto-immune paleo since October 2012. I only had one minor flare-up after an accidental exposure to I'm assuming gluten, it could have been white potato as well though. I knew very soon that something didn't agree with me and sure enough a minor breakout in my armpit. After your article and becoming more aware of what HS is I realize I have had some of these boils there before, never as painful as the ones down below though.

Thank you, thank you, thank you! I never would have known what this was and that I could control it with my diet. Thank you so much!"

—Barb

I came across you about two to three months ago, and read some articles that you had posted regarding this condition. Anyway just to let you know that I gave up eating potatoes about two to three months ago and the condition has cleared up (after sixteen years of having it). I still get the very odd small spot, which could be just a spot, but the main problem has gone away.

So thanks very much!

—Anonymous

The first time that I had read that HS might be due to a food allergy, I remember thinking, "Oh sure...." The best doctors in the world can't figure this thing out, and I am supposed to believe that I get these miserable lesions because of what I eat.

But after trying everything by the book ... antibiotics, topicals, washing with a specific soap, trying to de-stress my life, losing weight (I lost fifty pounds), and finally, the most invasive of all, surgical removal of tissue—I was no closer to a cure than when I started.

It was time for me to do the research. Articles, I read everything I could get my hands on. I read blog after blog and came up with some amazing information. In essence our bodies are screaming at us through the HS lesions. We have and are consuming a food group whether it be gluten or nightshades or dairy or eggs that are making our bodies attack themselves. Simple. Find out what the offending food is and remove it. Either by going to see a Naturopath for an IgE and an IeE food sensitivity test. Or if you financially aren't able to do that, then simply put yourself on a diet of protein, simple salads, and green vegetables. Once you have done that, introduce one food group at a time and wait to see if you flare. No flare. Wonderful ... now try another and another until you isolate the group that causes you to flare. Be vigilant at looking at labels.

If you are like me, you have lived with the fear of this disease on a day-to-day basis. You have kept yourself isolated for fear that someone might find out. The pain is so intolerable as is the stigma of this disease. But you can take your life back. You can be happy again. It is a process and it will take time and diligence. You deserve a chance at living a normal life. God be with you."

— Catherine

PUT YOUR MONEY WHERE YOUR MOUTH IS

It's amazing to me that the Western medical community is so clueless when it comes to HS. Take, for example, breast cancer. We ALL know what breast cancer is. Not that I am belittling the disease or the tenacity of its survivors, but if I have one more person ask me to donate to Breast Cancer Awareness, I am going to scream. We're all AWARE of breast cancer already. I can't be any MORE aware of it. Am I giving them money so that they can go into undeveloped areas of the world and tell people what breast cancer is? So that they can be aware of it too?

They're certainly not using the money we donate to run human trials on the effects of consuming unnatural chemicals and frankenfoods, or on the effects when these unnatural foods are removed from the diet. No, that would make too much sense and not enough money for Big Pharma.

And that's what it comes down to. A natural approach to autoimmune disease doesn't make any money for the doctors, the drug companies, and the medical industry. Until we rise up and prove to them that we can heal ourselves, our brothers and sisters will continue to be subjected to experimental drugs and butchering surgeries.

I have heard from people all over the world who are afflicted with HS. It's not an American problem. Yet, there is no awareness for HS. No funds, no campaigns for the cure, nothing. Your doctor may not even know what it is, but he will be happy to prescribe the latest experimental drug.

We need to come out of the closet, people. HS may not kill you, but I am certain that people have committed suicide because of it. I know this because there have been times I have wanted to kill myself. Times I have been so ashamed of the condition of my body that I just wanted it all to end. Times when I have been so frustrated with doctors and their lack of compassion, making me feel ashamed of myself, like it was MY FAULT, that I wanted to give up. Times when I got my hopes raised up so high that the latest drugs were going to cure me, and dashed lower than ever before when they actually made me worse.

And I'm one of the lucky ones! My HS wasn't even all that bad compared to some other folks.

Unlike breast cancer, we definitely need awareness about HS—especially within the medical and psychiatric communities, but also for our friends and families and for those who are suffering and don't even know what they have.

The next time someone asks you to donate money for a disease other than HS, ask yourself if that money is going to actually cure a disease or if it is simply going toward administrative costs for a campaign to raise awareness. Ask yourself (or the representative) who exactly is benefiting from any money you give. (Better yet, ask them what specific headway they've made toward a cure.)

If you have success with healing your HS because of this book (and I hope you do), please visit your doctor and tell her that a natural approach worked for you. Talk about your condition to others, start a blog, spread the word—there are too many of us out there who are still alone and searching for answers.

While I want to raise awareness, I also want to help people understand and find a solution for their HS. I personally am willing to give copies of this book at cost for distribution to doctor's offices and hospitals, especially within the military medical community, since I have been subjected to its incompetence my entire life. For more information, or if you know of a doctor that could benefit from reading this book, please contact me at PrimalGirl.com.

Remember that this is a life-long journey and struggle. There will be relapses and remission. Don't be too hard on yourself if you can't achieve perfection. It will take time for your body to heal and you can't be perfect all the time.

Wear your battle scars proudly, for they mark a time in your life when you gave your power away to an industry that didn't care. When you look at those scars, hold your head up high—you have taken that power back. You alone hold the key to your health and happiness. You can do this. Just take it one day at a time.

Tara Grant
September 9, 2013
Phoenix, Arizona

ACKNOWLEDGMENTS

I wish to thank Dr. Loren Cordain, author of *The Paleo Diet*, for first mentioning the connection between hidradenitis suppurativa and autoimmunity to me. He gave me the tools to forever change my life and health. I also wish to acknowledge my publisher Mark Sisson. Through his book, *The Primal Blueprint*, he was the first to introduce me to the Primal lifestyle and remains one of my biggest influences. He's changed the way I think, the way I play, and even the way I express myself.

To Robb Wolf, author of *The Paleo Solution*: you are one of the coolest guys I know. Thank you for helping me out during a time that I now know was a difficult time for you. Actually, thank you for helping me every single time I ask for help. I'm seriously in love with you. To Sarah Ballantyne: without your website, I would not understand half the science in this book. You are an incredible teacher and I am proud to know you. To Brad Kearns: thank you so much for including me in everything. I once promised I wouldn't let you down, and I hope I never do. To Tess McEnulty: if you hadn't emailed me that day, I wouldn't be where I am now. You changed my world, and I'm grateful.

To Jessica Taylor Tudzin, my amazing editor. Thank you for all the time, effort, and attention you spent making this book perfect, and for really giving a shit and getting who I am. A special thank you also goes to Caroline De Vita for the interior book design and its inspirational imagery. To Orleatha Smith, Mickey Trescott, and Brandon and Megan Keatley, who all contributed recipes to this book: your culinary creations are divine and make healing so much more enjoyable. To Kiley, Wendy, and everyone else who shared their stories and pictures: thank you for opening up and helping others.

And finally to my family. To my little brother Jeffy: thank you for seeing what I needed at a time I couldn't. If it weren't for you, I wouldn't have found this lifestyle when I needed it most. To my Mom and Dad: Thank you for being so supportive, and for making me feel loved, always. To my children, Taylor and Gibson: Thank you for making me realize my worth, and for being really great kids.

And to my husband, Derek: thank you for never giving up on me—even when I was at my worst—and for constantly building me up. You have given me the strength to resist potatoes. I love you.

APPENDIX A

HIGH FODMAP FRUITS:
- Apples
- Apricots
- Cherries
- Dates
- Figs
- Mango
- Nectarines
- Papaya
- Peaches
- Pears
- Plum
- Watermelon
- Avocado
- Dried Fruit

HIGH FODMAP VEGETABLES:
- Anise/fennel root
- Artichoke
- Asparagus
- Beets
- Broccoli
- Brussel sprouts
- Cabbage
- Cauliflower
- Celery
- Garlic
- Leeks
- Mushrooms
- Okra
- Onion/shallot
- Snow/sugar snap peas

FODMAP is an acronym for:
Fermentable, Oligo-, Di-, Mono-saccharides and Polyols.

Please note that even the experts disagree on different high FODMAP foods; you should keep a journal to see which foods give you intestinal upset, and which ones don't.

APPENDIX B

DAY 56
WEEK 8

DATE
/ /

1 - 10 SCORE

Energy:	"Big M":	Health:	Mood:	Stress:

DIET   Success Score:_____

DATA

Weight:	Fat %:	x1: _____	x2: _____

Meals:_____

MACRONUTRIENT CALCULATIONS

Carbs:	Protein:	Fat:	Calories:

_____

_____

_____

_____

_____

_____

_____

Snacks:_____

_____

Comments:_____

_____

_____

_____

PRIMAL LIFESTYLE   Success Score:_____

Sleep (1-10):_____ Comments:_____
Sun (1-10):_____ Comments:_____
Play (1-10):_____ Comments:_____
Brain (1-10):_____ Comments:_____
Move (1-10):_____ Comments:_____

PERSONAL

Comments:_____

_____

_____

EXERCISE   Success Score:_____   Effort Score:_____

Workout:_____

Location:_____   Duration:_____

Exercise 1:_____ Weight:_____ Reps/Time:_____ Set 2:_____ Set 3:_____

Exercise 2:_____ Weight:_____ Reps/Time:_____ Set 2:_____ Set 3:_____

Exercise 3:_____ Weight:_____ Reps/Time:_____ Set 2:_____ Set 3:_____

Exercise 4:_____ Weight:_____ Reps/Time:_____ Set 2:_____ Set 3:_____

Exercise 5:_____ Weight:_____ Reps/Time:_____ Set 2:_____ Set 3:_____

Exercise 6:_____ Weight:_____ Reps/Time:_____ Set 2:_____ Set 3:_____

Comments:_____

_____

_____

_____

_____

Workout:_____

Location:_____   Distance:_____   Duration:_____

Comments:_____

_____

_____

_____

_____

SUMMARY

Tomorrow:_____

This Week:_____   This Month:_____

Wins:_____

Challenges:_____

Comments:_____

_____

_____

_____

_____

One Word   Success Score (1-10)

Sample journal pages courtesy of Mark Sisson, *The Primal Blueprint 90-Day Journal.*

RESOURCES

If you still have questions, don't worry. You can get all the information you need if you just take the time to find it. The Internet is an amazing resource, and you can find most of the stuff you need—like recipes, shopping tips, and detailed information on specific subjects relevant to you—for free.

There are resources that are raising awareness and research specifically for HS and building communities online for those of us afflicted. Please stop by their websites and check them out. It will help them to know that you exist and that they have your support. Be sure to also check out the Primal and Paleo communities online. They are a fantastic resource for support, recipes, and information.

Realizing that you alone hold the key to reclaiming your health is incredibly empowering. Take back your power and become an advocate for your health today!

HS Specific Resources

PRIMALGIRL HS FORUMS
By the time this book is published, the forum on my website will be live. I would like to use it primarily as a resource for people who have read this book and who are looking for support but who know what it will evolve into. Membership will be free and confidential. I'll also be posting some of my favorite recipes. PrimalGirl.com/forums

HIDRADENITIS SUPPURATIVA USA
A support group and forum for HS patients. Contains links to medical studies, information, and the latest research into HS. Members may connect with other members for support, post pictures, and blog about their experiences. HS-USA.webs.com

THE HS DIET CONNECTION
A Facebook support group that recognizes the connection between HS and diet. It's a closed group in order to keep your identity and information confidential, but you can request membership on the main page. Facebook.com/Groups/HSandGlutenFree

HS DIET LOG

A handy (and free) resource created by the owner of The HS and Diet Connection Facebook page. This website allows you to track your flare-ups, what and when you ate, and even includes factors like the humidity level, flare-up severity, and your stress level. Handy for those of us who are always on the go. HSDiet.com

PUBMED

The latest research studies on HS are posted on this site. Once you've learned a few key terms, you should be able to navigate this site and read the latest scientific findings for yourself. Invaluable if you are considering medication, surgery, or supplements. Just search for "hidradenitis suppurativa" and sift through the results. If you're unsure what the studies are saying (most use technical terms and reference the latest in drug options and surgery), forward them to a naturopath or doctor and ask for an explanation. PubMed.com

KILEY MACLEOD

Kiley's story is featured in this book. She has been suffering from HS for several years and is in Stage III. Her blog features interviews with doctors, up-to-date information on the latest medical breakthroughs, and detailed personal information. Kiley has been through several rounds of HS surgery and is a great resource for those of you considering it. She is also on a (mostly) Paleolithic diet and has identified several food triggers. NotDying.wordpress.com

HS HOMEMADE SOLUTIONS

A fellow HS sufferer has designed a line of products specifically for people with the disease. Sheryl makes cotton sanitary pads that don't cause flare-ups, rice bags for either hot or cold compresses, and other fabulous homemade products useful for HS. Facebook.com/HSHome-madeSolutionsBySheryl

Autoimmunity Experts

Dr. Sarah Ballantyne, Ph.D., B.Sc., ThePaleoMom.com
Dr. Loren Cordain, Ph.D., ThePaleoDiet.com
Chris Kresser, L.Ac, ChrisKresser.com

Learn How to Cook

THE RELUCTANT GOURMET

A cooking website for people that don't know how to cook. Learn how to separate an egg, make a simple dressing, and cut up a chicken. Free videos are included on the site.
ReluctantGourmet.com/tips-guides/cooking-videos

EPICURIOUS

A website full of different techniques and recipes to have you cooking like a Master Chef in no time. Epicurious.com/video/technique-videos

BATCH COOKERY

Learn the skills you need to be able to cook 160 meals in under six hours—how to shop, prepare, and store all that food you're making, as well. Batch cooking (or being a super cook) saves time, money, and frees you up to do other things. BatchCookery.com

AMERICA'S TEST KITCHEN

This site gets super scientific about specific techniques. Find out exactly which cookware you should use when, including which foods are best for non-stick skillets versus regular pans. America's Test Kitchen actually runs scientific tests and delivers the results to you.
TrueFire.com/cooktv/

Helpful Books

RECIPE BOOKS

Cooking Against the Grain, Orleatha Smith
Eat Like s Dinosaur: Recipe and Guidebook for Gluten-Free Kids,
   The Paleo Parents
Paleo Breakfasts and Lunches On the Go, Diana Rodgers
Paleo Cooking from Elana's Pantry, Elana Amsterdam
Practical Paleo, Diane Sanfilippo
Primal Cravings, Megan McCullough Keatley and Brandon Keatley
Real Food Fermentation, Alex Lewin
The Autoimmune Paleo Cookbook, Mickey Trescott
   (Use code **DefeatHS** for 25 percent off at Autoimmune-Paleo.com!)
The Ice Dream Cookbook: Dairy-Free Ice Cream Alternatives,
   Rachel Albert-Matesz
The Paleo Approach Cookbook, Sarah Ballantyne (2014)
The Primal Blueprint Cookbook, Mark Sisson with Jennifer Meier

MISCELLANEOUS BOOKS

Becoming a Supple Leopard, Kelly Starrett with Glen Cordoza
Breaking the Vicious Cycle: Intestinal Health Through Diet,
   Elaine Gottschall
Lights Out: Sleep, Sugar, and Survival, T.S. Wiley with Bent Formby
Modern Cave Girl: Paleo Living in the Concrete Jungle, Liz Wolfe
Nourishing Traditions, Sally Fallon with Mary G. Enig
Paleo Fitness, Darryl Edwards with Brett Stewart and Jason Warner
Perfect Health Diet, Paul Jaminet and Shou-Ching Jaminet
Paleo Manifesto, John Durant
Primal Moms Look Good Naked, Peggy Emch
Rich Food, Poor Food, Jayson and Mira Calton
The Modern No-Nonsense Guide to Paleo, Alison Golden
The Paleo Approach: Reverse Autoimmune Disease, Heal Your Body,
   Sarah Ballantyne
Wheat Belly, William Davis
Why We Get Fat, Gary Taubes

Autoimmune Paleo Recipes Online

A quick Google search for "autoimmune Paleo recipes" will turn up thousands of solutions for your dinner tonight. If you'd like somewhere specific to start, here are some of my favorite sites.

Diane Sanfilippo (Balanced Bites): BalancedBites.com
Elana Amsterdam (Elana's Pantry): ElanasPantry.com
Michelle Tam (NomNomPaleo): NomNomPaleo.com
Mickey Trescott (Autoimmune Paleo): AutoimmunePaleo.com
Orleatha Smith (Level Health and Nutrition): LVLHealth.com
Sarah Ballantyne (The Paleo Mom): ThePaleoMom.com
Stacy Toth (The Paleo Parents): PaleoParents.com

Paleo/Primal Resources

Loren Cordain: Loren Cordain PhD, is an American scientist who specializes in the fields of nutrition and exercise physiology. He is an advocate of the Paleolithic diet and does research into Paleolithic nutrition. He has written numerous peer-reviewed articles on the subject as well as many popular books including *The Paleo Diet*. He is currently a tenured professor in the Department of Health and Exercise at Colorado State University. Dr. Cordain is well versed in hidradenitis suppurativa. ThePaleoDiet.com

Robb Wolf: Robb Wolf is a former research biochemist and the author of the New York Times bestseller *The Paleo Solution—The Original Human Diet*. Robb was a student of Prof. Loren Cordain and has transformed the lives of thousands of people around the world. He can be reached through his blog and heard weekly on his top ranked iTunes podcast. Robbwolf.com

Mark Sisson: Mark Sisson is an American fitness author and blogger and a former distance runner, triathlete, and Ironman competitor who healed his IBS through removing grains and other Neolithic foods from his diet. He has written several books including *The Primal Blueprint* and *The Primal Connection*. Sisson also blogs at his website Mark's Daily Apple and coordinates annual Primal Conventions and Primal Transformation Seminars nationwide. MarksDailyApple.com and PrimalBlueprint.com

Nora Gedgaudas: Nora Gedgaudas is one of the world's leading experts on Paleolithic nutrition and author of the international bestselling book *Primal Body, Primal Mind: Beyond the Paleo Diet for Total Health and a Longer Life*. She maintains a private practice in Portland, Oregon, as both a Certified Nutritional Therapist (CNT) and a Board-certified Clinical Neurofeedback Specialist (CNS). PrimalBody-PrimalMind. com

Chris Kresser: Chris Kresser is a licensed acupuncturist and practitioner of integrative medicine with a private practice in Berkeley, California. He is the author of *The Personal Paleo Code*, *The Healthy Baby Code* and *The Paleo Meal Plan Generator*. Chris is an expert in autoimmune issues and is a wealth of information, which he shares regularly on his blog and on his top-rated podcast. ChrisKresser.com

Diane Sanfilippo: Diane Sanfilippo is a Holistic Nutritionist specializing in Paleo nutrition, blood sugar regulation, food allergies, and intolerances and digestive health. She is the author of *Practical Paleo* and *The 21-Day Sugar Detox* program as well as the co-host of the *Balanced Bites* podcast on iTunes. *Practical Paleo* is both a science book, explaining the fundamentals of Paleo, and a cookbook with many autoimmune friendly recipes. BalancedBites.com

The Ancestral Health Symposium: Started in 2011, this annual event has been dubbed "The Woodstock of Natural Medicine." Doctors, researchers, scientists and laymen from around the world travel to AHS to share their latest findings and to learn more about ancestral health and evolutionary biology. In order to make this information accessible to everyone, the Ancestral Health Society posts videos and show notes from the Symposium each year. AncestralHealth.org

Paleo Physicians Network and **Primal Docs:** two websites dedicated to finding you a paleo-friendly physician. These doctors take an evolutionary approach to health, nutrition, medicine, and lifestyle. Find a paleo-friendly doctor or naturopath near you if you need extra help or if you want testing done. PaleoPhysiciansNetwork.com and PrimalDocs.com

The Paleo Foundation: a non-profit organization whose mission is to strengthen, unify, and further the paleo movement. The Paleo Foundation accomplishes this mission by offering community outreach programs, events, and grants that serve to educate and promote growth within the paleo community and making farm and food labeling services available that protect the integrity of the word "paleo." PaleoFoundation.org

Sourcing Ingredients

FARMERS MARKETS AND CO-OPS
Local CSA Farmers Market Directory, LocalHarvest.org
Organic Consumers Association, OrganicConsumers.org/foodcoops.htm

GRASS-FED FARMS
Eat Wild, EatWild.com
Tendergrass Farms, GrassFedBeef.org

MEAT, FISH, AND PRODUCE DELIVERY
Brandon Natural Beef, BrandonNaturalBeef.com
Diestel Turkey, DiestelTurkey.com
North Star Bison, NorthStarBison.com
Slanker's, TexasGrassfedBeef.com
The Fruit Guys, FruitGuys.com
Thompson River Ranch, ThompsonRiverRanch.com
Topline Foods, TopLineFoods.com
US Wellness Meats, GrasslandBeef.com
Vital Choice, VitalChoice.com
Wild Alaskan Salmon Company, Seabeef.com
Wild Pacific Salmon, WildPacificSalmon.com

MISCELLANEOUS INGREDIENTS
Grass-fed Gelatin
Great Lakes, GreatLakesGelatin.com

Grass-fed Ghee
Pure Indian Foods, PureIndianFoods.com

Coconut Oil and Shortening
Spectrum, SpectrumOrganics.com

Grass-fed Beef Jerky
Nick's Sticks, Nicks-Sticks.com
Primal Pacs, PrimalPacs.com
Slant Shack Jerky, SlantShackJerky.com
Steve's Paleo Goods, StevesPaleoGoods.com
The New Primal, TheNewPrimal.com

Skincare Products
Radiant Life, RadiantLifeCatalog.com

Stevia
Sweetleaf, SweetLeaf.com

GLOSSARY

Abscess: a localized collection of pus surrounded by inflamed tissue. It is a defensive reaction of the tissue to prevent the spread of infectious materials to other parts of the body.

Acne conglobata: a subtype of Follicular Occulsion Syndrome.

Acne inversa: another name for hidradenitis suppurativa. The name implies that HS is acne that is "inversed" or below the skin.

Adrenocorticotropic hormone (ACTH): a hormone secreted by the anterior pituitary gland. It is produced in response to biological stress (along with it's precursor corticotrophin-releasing hormone). Its main effects are increased production and release of corticosteroids like cortisol.

Adjuvant: a pharmacological or immunological agent that modifies the effect of other agents, such as a drug or vaccine. Adjuvants are often included in vaccines to enhance the recipient's immune response.

Aldosterone: a steroid hormone in the mineral corticosteroid family. It is produced by the outer section of the adrenal cortex in the adrenal gland, and causes the conservation of sodium, the secretion of potassium, increased water retention, and increased blood pressure.

Alkaloid: a group of naturally occurring chemical compounds that contain mostly basic nitrogen atoms. Alkaloids are produced by a large variety of organisms, including bacteria, fungi, plants and animals. Many alkaloids are toxic to other organisms. They often have pharmacological effects and can be used as medications and recreational drugs. Examples are the local anesthetic and stimulant cocaine, the psychedelic psilocin, the stimulants caffeine and nicotine, the analgesic morphine, the antibacterial berberine, the anticancer compound vincristine, the antihypertension agent reserpine, the vasodilator vincamine, and the antimalarial drug quinine.

Anabolic hormones: opposite of catabolic hormones. Anabolic metabolic processes build up organs and tissues, increase growth and differentiation of cells, and increase body size. Anabolic hormones include testosterone, human growth hormone, and insulin.

Androgen: a male sex hormone. The primary and most well known androgen is testosterone.

Antinutrients: compounds that interfere with the absorption of nutrients. Some are more detrimental than others.

Lectins appear in high concentrations in cereal grains, beans, seeds, nuts and potatoes. They are proteins that are part of the plant's natural defense system. Adverse effects on humans may include nutritional deficiencies, immune or allergic reactions, gastrointestinal distress, and leaky gut. Many lectins can be disabled by soaking, sprouting, and fermenting.

Phytic acid and *phytates* have a strong binding affect on minerals such as calcium, magnesium, iron, copper, and zinc. This makes the minerals unavailable for absorption in the intestines.

Antibacterial: an agent that inhibits bacterial growth or kills bacteria.

Antibiotic: a substance designed to prevent, inhibit, or destroy harmful bacteria and fungus. Problem is, they also kill off beneficial microorganisms, often causing diarrhea, allergies, and development of drug-resistant strains of the targeted microorganisms.

Antibody: a large Y-shaped protein used by the immune system to identify and neutralize *antigens,* or foreign objects such as bacteria and viruses. The production of antibodies is the main function of the immune system.

Antifungal: an agent that inhibits fungal growth or kills fungi.

Antimicrobial: an agent that kills microorganisms or inhibits their growth.

Apocrine glands: also known as sweat glands and located at the junction of the skin and the subcutaneous fat. In humans, apocrine sweat glands are found only in certain locations of the body: the armpits, areola and nipples of the breast, the ear canal, eyelids, wings of the nostril, perianal region, and some parts of the external genitalia. The rest of the body is covered by *eccrine sweat glands*. The apocrine glands become involved in HS when there is intense inflammation in the body, or if a patient is in stage III.

Autoimmunity: the failure of an organism to recognize its own parts as *self*, which allows an immune response against its own cells and tissues.

Autoimmune disease: a disease that results from an inappropriate immune response.

Bio-identical: a term referring to anything that is identical (on a molecular level) to what our body produces. Bio-identical is mostly used to refer to hormones, but can also be used to refer to proteins or other molecules that the human body recognizes as its own.

Boil: bumpy, red, pus-filled lumps around a hair follicle that are tender, warm, and very painful. They range from pea-sized to golf ball-sized. Sometimes referred to as *furuncles*, boils are essentially an infection of the hair follicle and are the primary symptom of HS.

Candida albicans: a type of fungus that grows both as yeast and as filamentous cells.

Carbuncle: individual boils clustered together.

Casein: The main protein found in milk.

Catabolic hormones: opposite of anabolic hormones. Catabolic metabolic processes break down organs and tissues, reduce growth and differentiation of cells and decrease body size. Catabolic hormones include cortisol, glucagon, adrenaline, cytokines, and melatonin.

Circulatory system: a network of blood vessels and lymphatic vessels that transport nutrients from the gut to other areas of the body.

Cortisol: a steroid hormone produced in the adrenal cortex and released in response to stress. Its primary function is to increase blood sugar, suppress the immune system, and to aid in fat, protein, and carbohydrate metabolism.

Corticotropin-releasing hormone (CRH): a peptide hormone and neurotransmitter involved in the stress response. Its main function is the stimulation of ACTH.

Cytokines: Greek for cell ("cyto-") and movement ("-kinos"), cytokines are small messenger molecules used for cell signaling. Cytokines make up a large and diverse family of regulators produced throughout the body and are involved in several developmental processes that are crucial in immune functioning. Some of their effects are systemic (body wide) and some are local.

Dehydroepiandrosterone (DHEA): a steroid hormone produced in the adrenal glands, the gonads, and the brain. DHEA is the precursor for testosterone and estrogen.

Dendritic cells: a type of immune cell. Their main function is to process antigen material and present it to other cells of the immune system.

Digestive enzymes: enzymes that break down food for absorption by the body. Digestive enzymes are found in saliva and the digestive tract.

Diseases of Civilization (DOCs): Sometimes referred to as lifestyle diseases or diseases of longevity, DOCs are diseases that appear to increase in frequency as countries become more industrialized and people live longer. They can include Alzheimer's disease, asthma, cancer, type II diabetes, heart disease, metabolic syndrome, stroke, depression, obesity and others. Studies have linked DOCs with a Western lifestyle and diet and have shown that early hunter-gatherer societies were virtually free of all the aforementioned conditions.

Dissecting cellulitis: a subtype of follicular occlusion syndrome. This is a scalp condition consisting of large nodules and cysts filled with pus that lead to scarring and hair loss.

Dysbiosis: also called dysbacteriosis, dysbiosis is a condition that results in microbial imbalances on or inside the body. It is most prominent in the digestive tract or on the skin but can occur on any exposed surface or mucous membrane such as the vagina, lungs, mouth, nose, sinuses, ears, nails, or eyes. Imbalances in the intestinal microbiome are associated with bowel inflammation, chronic fatigue syndrome, inflammatory bowel disease and irritable bowel syndrome.

Enterocytes: simple cells that line the small intestines and colon. They are responsible for the absorption of water and the uptake of sugars, proteins, and fats. Enterocytes are also responsible for vitamin B12, sodium, calcium, magnesium, and iron uptake. They can be damaged by various antinutrients such as lectins. When this happens, vitamins and minerals are not properly absorbed by the body.

Estrogen: a steroid hormone present in both men and women. Estrogen is the primary female sex hormone.

Fistula: an abnormal connection or passageway between two organs or vessels that normally do not connect. In severe HS, fistula may form connecting HS lesions together. It is generally a disease condition, but a fistula may be surgically created for therapeutic reasons. A *blind fistula* has one open end, a *complete fistula* has both external and internal openings and an *incomplete fistula* has an external skin opening that does not connect to any internal organ.

Follicular occlusion syndrome: a group of inflammatory skin diseases affecting the hair follicles. The presentation of symptoms is dependent on the subtype of the condition. They are as follows: hidradenitis suppurativa, acne conglobata, dissecting cellulitis, and pilonidal disease.

Fungus: a member of a large group of organisms that includes microorganisms such as yeasts, molds, and mushrooms. Plural: fungi.

Gliadin: a protein present in wheat and several other cereals within the grass genus *Triticum* such as rye and barley. Gliadins and *glutens* are the two main components of the gluten fraction of the wheat seed. Gliadin is the soluble aspect of it, while glutenin is insoluble. There are three main types of gliaden (α, Y, and ω). It is possible to be intolerant or even allergic to gliaden. Some research has found that gliaden affects the human brain.

Gluten: a protein present in wheat and several other cereals within the grass genus *Triticum* such as rye and barley. Gluten gives elasticity to dough, helps it rise and keep it's shape and often makes the final product chewy. However, gluten is directly responsible for Celiac disease and many people are intolerant to it. Gluten is in all baked goods containing wheat and may also be found in some cosmetics, hair products, and other dermatological preparations.

Glycoalkaloid: an alkaloid plus a sugar molecule. Glycoalkaloids are a family of poisons found commonly in the nightshade plant species. There are several glycoalkaloids that are potentially toxic. They are poorly absorbed by the gastrointestinal tract but can cause gastrointestinal irritation. The alkaloid portion of a glycoalkaloid can be absorbed and is believed to be responsible for observed nervous system signs. Glycoalkaloids are bitter tasting and produce a burning irritation in the back of the mouth and side of the tongue when eaten.

Glycoside: in chemistry, a glycoside is a molecule in which a sugar is bound to a non-carbohydrate molecule.

Gut barrier: see *Intestinal wall.*

Gut flora: bacteria that live in the digestive tracts of humans and animals. The largest reservoir of human flora. In this context, gut is synonymous with *intestinal,* and *flora* with *microbiota* and *microflora*; the word *microbiome* is also in use.

Gut integrity: whether or not the intestine is leaking, damaged, or inflamed.

Hair follicle: Found underneath the skin, a hair follicle essentially produces a hair. In Stage I and II HS, the hair follicle becomes inflamed. It is then clogged with sebum or keratin and produces a painful boil underneath the skin. Other structures associated with the hair follicle include the sebaceous glands, and the apocrine sweat glands.

Hypha: a long, branching filamentous structure of a fungus, like the roots of a plant. Plural: *hyphae*.

IBD: Inflammatory Bowel Disease.

IBS: Irritable Bowel Syndrome.

Immune cells: Cells of the immune system, including *cytokines*, *eicosanoids* and *leukocytes*.

Immune response: When the immune system is activated.

Immune system: a system of biological structures and processes within an organism that protects against disease. To function properly, an immune system must detect a wide variety of agents, from viruses to parasitic worms and distinguish them from the organism's own healthy tissue. Disorders of the immune system can result in autoimmune disease, inflammatory disease, and cancer.

Incision and drainage: Incision and drainage and clinical lancing are minor surgical procedures to release pus or pressure built up under the skin, such as from an abscess or boil. It is performed by treating the area with an antiseptic and then making a small incision to puncture the skin. This allows the pus fluid to escape by draining out of the incision. Large abscesses require the insertion of a drainage tube. Many HS patients who have had incision and drainage report that their wound is slow to heal or never heals at all. Incision and drainage is often abbreviated as "I&D" or "IND" by medical professionals, or referred to as *lancing*.

Inflammation: part of the complex biological response of tissues to harmful stimuli, such as pathogens, damaged cells, or irritants. The classic signs of acute inflammation are pain, heat, redness, swelling, and loss of function. Inflammation is a protective attempt to remove the harmful stimuli and to initiate the healing process. Inflammation is not synonymous with infection, even in cases where inflammation is caused by an infection.

Insulin: a peptide hormone, produced by the pancreas. Insulin regulates carbohydrate and fat metabolism in the body and causes the cells in the liver, skeletal muscles, and fat tissue to absorb glucose from the blood to be used for energy, or stored for later. In the liver and skeletal muscles, glucose is stored as *glycogen*, and in fat cells it is stored as *triglycerides*.

Insulin index: a measure used to quantify the typical insulin response to various foods. The index is similar to the Glycemic Index and Glycemic Load, but rather than relying on blood glucose levels, the Insulin Index is based upon blood insulin levels. Certain foods can cause an insulin response despite there being no carbohydrates present, and some foods cause a disproportionate insulin response relative to their carbohydrate load, so the Insulin Index may be more useful to people suffering from diabetes, insulin resistance, and metabolic syndrome than the Glycemic Index.

Insulin resistance (IR): a condition in which cells fail to respond to the normal actions of the hormone insulin. The body produces insulin but is unable to use it effectively. Glucose is automatically stored as fat instead of used for energy, producing fatigue, constant hunger, and obesity. Beta cells in the pancreas increase the production of insulin, further contributing to high levels in the body. This often remains undetected and can contribute to type 2 diabetes.

Insulinemic: something which elicits an excess of insulin to be produced and released.

Intestinal permeability: see *Leaky Gut*.

Intestinal wall: Also referred to as *Gut Barrier*. The wall of the intestine, through which nutrients pass.

Intestine: In human anatomy, the intestine (or bowel, hose, or gut) is the segment of the alimentary canal extending from the pyloric sphincter of the stomach to the anus. In humans and other mammals, the intestine consists of two segments, the small intestine and the large intestine. In humans, the small intestine is further subdivided into the duodenum, jejunum, and ileum, while the large intestine is subdivided into the cecum and colon.

Leaky gut: A state in which the intestine is leaking, damaged, or inflamed. Molecules which normally cannot pass through the intestinal wall are able to pass through and travel into the bloodstream. See the chapter on *Leaky Gut* for more detailed information.

Lectins: see *Antinutrients.*

Lesion: an abnormality or damage in the tissue of an organism, usually caused by disease or trauma.

Leukopenia: a decrease in the number of white blood cells (leukocytes) found in the blood, which places individuals at increased risk of infection. Someone with this condition is said to be *leukopenic. Neutropenia*, a subtype of leucopenia, refers to a decrease in the number of circulating neutrophil granulocytes, the most abundant white blood cells. The terms leucopenia and neutropenia may occasionally be used interchangeably, as the neutrophil count is the most important indicator of infection risk.

Leukocytes: White blood cells. Leukocytes are cells of the immune system involved in defending the body against both infectious disease and foreign materials.

Lymphatic system: part of the circulatory system, made up of a network of conduits called *lymphatic vessels* that carry a clear liquid called *lymph* towards the heart. The primary function of the lymphatic system is to provide an accessory route for excess filtered plasma to get returned to the blood. Lymphatic organs such as the tonsils, spleen, thymus, and bone marrow, play an important part in the immune system.

Lymphocyte: a kind of white blood cell in the immune system, specifically the adaptive immune system. They include natural killer cells (NK cells), T-cells, and B-cells.

Lysozyme: an enzyme that damages bacterial cell walls. Lysozyme is abundant in a number of secretions, such as tears, saliva, human milk, and mucus. Large amounts of lysozyme can be found in egg white.

Macrophage: versatile cells that play many roles in the body. As scavengers, they rid the body of worn-out cells and other debris. Along with *dendritic cells*, they are foremost among the cells that "present" antigen, a crucial role in initiating an immune response. As secretory cells, macrophages are vital to the regulation of immune responses and the development of inflammation.

Metabolic syndrome: a combination of the medical disorders that, when occurring together, increase the risk of developing cardiovascular disease and diabetes. Some studies have shown the prevalence in the USA to be an estimated 25 percent of the population and the prevalence increases with age. Metabolic syndrome is also known as metabolic syndrome X, cardiometabolic syndrome, syndrome X, insulin resistance, insulin resistance syndrome, Reaven's syndrome and CHAOS (in Australia). It is caused by eating too many carbohydrates over a long period of time. Some of the diseases associated with metabolic syndrome include type 2 diabetes, hyperuricemia and gout, PCOS, and fatty liver leading to NAFLD. Signs and symptoms of metabolic syndrome include, but are not limited to, the following: high blood pressure, central obesity, decreased HDL cholesterol, elevated triglycerides, insulin resistance, and fasting hyperglycemia.

Metabolism: the set of life-sustaining chemical transformations within the cells of living organisms that allow them to grow and reproduce, maintain their structure and respond to their environment. Metabolism also refers to digestion and the transport of substances into and between different cells.

Microorganism: Also known as a microbe, a microorganism is a microscopic organism, which may consist of a single cell or more than one cell. Either way, you can't see it with the naked eye.

Mucous membrane: an epithelium lining involved in absorption and secretion. Mucous membranes line cavities that are exposed to the external environment, chiefly the respiratory, digestive, and urogenital tracts. They are at several places contiguous with the skin: at the nostrils, the lips of the mouth, the eyelids, the ears, the genital area, and the anus. The sticky, thick fluid they excrete is called *mucus*, which traps pathogens in the body, preventing any further activities of diseases. Mucous membranes each have their own distinctive flora, which help to maintain balance and halt disease.

Mycotoxin: a toxin produced by molds.

Neolithic: a period in the development of human technology, beginning about 10,200 BC, commencing with the beginning of farming and agriculture. It marks the progression of behavioral and cultural characteristics and changes, including the use of wild and domestic crops and of domesticated animals.

Nightshades: an economically important family of flowering plants called *Solanaceae*. The family ranges from herbs to trees and includes a number of important agricultural crops, medicinal plants, spices, weeds, and ornamentals. Many members of the family contain potent alkaloids and some are highly toxic. Many cultures eat nightshades—in some cases as a staple food. Because of the antinutrients and the toxins they contain, nightshades can be very aggravating to autoimmune disorders. See also *Alkaloids*.

NSAIDs: Nonsteroidal anti-inflammatory drugs are a class of drugs that provide fever reducing and anti-inflammatory effects. They are non-addictive and non-narcotic. The most prominent members of this group of drugs are aspirin, ibuprofen, and naproxen, all of which are available over the counter in most countries. NSAIDs can cause leaky gut.

Nutrient: a chemical that an organism needs to live and grow, or a substance used in an organism's metabolism which must be taken in from its environment. Nutrients are used to build and repair tissues, regulate body processes, and are converted to and used as energy.

Paleolithic: a prehistoric period of human history distinguished by the development of the most primitive stone tools and covers roughly 99 percent of human technological prehistory. It extends from the earliest known use of stone tools, approximately 2.6 million years ago, to the end of the Pleistocene around ten thousand years ago.

Parasite: an organism that benefits at the expense of another, the *host*. *Parasitism* is a non-mutual relationship between organisms.

Pathogen: a microorganism that causes disease in its host. The host may be an animal (including humans), a plant, or even another microorganism. The pathogen may be a virus, parasite, bacterium, prion (misfolded protein), or fungus.

Peptides: short chains of amino acid monomers linked by peptide (amide) bonds.

Perifolliculitis capitis abscedens et suffodiens: see *dissecting cellulitis*.

Phytohaemagglutinin (PHA): a lectin found in plants, especially legumes. It is found in the highest concentrations in uncooked red kidney beans and white kidney beans (also known as cannellini) and is also found in lower quantities in many other types of green beans and other common beans, as well as broad beans and fava beans. It has a number of physiological effects and is used in medical research. In high doses, it is a toxin.

Phytates (Phytic Acid): see *Antinutrients*.

Pilonidal disease: a subtype of follicular occlusion syndrome. Pilonidal disease is a chronic skin problem found most often in the sacrococcygeal region. This is the cleft between the buttocks, just below the base of the spine.

Pilonidal sinus: a subtype of follicular occlusion syndrome, in which a sinus tract forms at the base of the spine. In most cases, this tract fills with nests of hair, hence the name pilonidal ("pilus" meaning hair, and "nidal" meaning nest). A pilonidal sinus may become infected, creating a *pilonidal abscess*.

Prebiotics: non-digestible food ingredients that stimulate the growth and/or activity of bacteria in the digestive system in ways claimed to be beneficial to health.

Precursor: in biochemistry, the term precursor is used to refer to a chemical compound preceding another in a metabolic pathway. For example, cortisol is made from progesterone. It can be said that progesterone is the *precursor* to cortisol.

Probiotics: live microorganisms that may confer a health benefit on the host.

Progesterone: a steroid hormone involved in the female menstrual cycle, pregnancy, and embryogenesis of humans and other species.

Prostaglandins: a subclass of *eicosanoids*, a type of immune cell.

Proteins: large biological molecules consisting of one or more chains of amino aicds. Proteins perform a vast array of functions within living organisms, including catalyzing metabolic reactions, replicating DNA, responding to stimuli, and transporting molecules from one location to another.

Pyridoxine glucoside: (also known as pyridoxine-5'-ß-D-glucoside). A major source of vitamin B6 in *plant-derived* foods. It partially impairs the absorption and metabolic utilization of co-ingested non-glycosylated forms of vitamin B6, like those found in meat. Lack of pyridoxine may lead to anemia, nerve damage, seizures, skin problems, and sores in the mouth.

Remission: the state of absence of disease activity in patients with a chronic illness, with the possibility of return of disease activity.

Saponin: a glycoside with a distinct foaming characteristic. Some saponins resemble human hormones and are able to weakly mimic them in the human body.

Sebaceous cyst: a term that loosely refers to either *epidermal cysts* or *pilar cysts*. Because an epidermal cyst originates in the epidermis and a pilar cyst originates from hair follicles, by definition, neither type of cyst is strictly a sebaceous cyst. The name is regarded as a misnomer as the fatty, white, semi-solid material in both these types of cysts is not sebum, but rather keratin. Furthermore, under the microscope, neither cyst contains sebaceous glands. In practice, however, the terms are often used interchangeably. True sebaceous cysts are rare and are known as *steatocystomas* or, if multiple, as *steatocystoma multiplex*.

Sex hormone-binding globulin (SHBG): a glycoprotein (protein and sugar) that binds to sex hormones, specifically androgens and estrogens. Other steroid hormones such as progesterone, cortisol, and other corticosteroids are bound by *transcortin*.

Standard American Diet (SAD): Also called the Western Pattern Diet, the Western dietary pattern, or the meat-sweet diet, SAD is a dietary habit chosen by many people in some developed countries and increasingly in developing countries. It is characterized by high intakes of red meat, sugary desserts, high-fat foods, and refined grains. It also typically contains dairy products, high sugar drinks and high intakes of processed foods.

Steroid hormones: a steroid that acts as a hormone. Steroid hormones, or *sterones,* can be grouped into five groups by the receptors to which they bind: *glucocorticoids* (cortisol), *mineralcorticoids* (aldosterone), *androgens* (testosterone), *estrogens* (estrogen) and *progestogens* (progesterone). Vitamin D derivatives are a sixth closely related hormone system, though they are technically sterols rather than steroids. Steroid hormones help control metabolism, inflammation, immune functions, salt and water balance, development of sexual characteristics, and the ability to withstand illness and injury

Subcutaneous: beneath the skin.

T-helper cells: a sub-group of lymphocytes, a type of white blood cell, that play an important role in the immune system, particularly in the adaptive immune system. They help the activity of other immune cells by releasing T-cell cytokines.

Testosterone: a steroid hormone from the androgen group, primarily secreted in the testes in men and the ovaries in women, although small amounts are also secreted by the adrenal glands. Testosterone is the principal male sex hormone.

Tight junctions: Tight junctions, or *zonula occludens*, are the closely associated areas of two cells whose membranes join together forming a virtually impermeable barrier to fluid.

Toxin: a poisonous substance produced within living cells or organisms; man-made substances created by artificial processes are thus excluded. Toxins can be small molecules, peptides, or proteins that are capable of causing disease on contact with or absorption by body tissues. Toxins vary greatly in their severity, ranging from usually minor and acute (bee sting) to almost immediately deadly (botulinum toxin.)

Trigger: a particular food or substance that results in a flare-up of your autoimmune condition.

Verneuil's disease: another name for hidradenitis suppurativa.

Villi: Singular: *villus*. Plural: *villi*. Intestinal villus refers to any one of the small, finger-shaped outgrowths of the epithelial lining of the wall of the intestine. Clusters of projections are referred as intestinal villi.

Virus: a small infectious agent that can replicate only inside the living cells of an organism. Viruses can infect all types of organisms, from animals and plants to bacteria.

Wheat germ agglutinin (WGA): a lectin that protects wheat from insects, yeast, and bacteria.

Yeast: microorganisms classified in the Fungi kingdom, with over
1,500 species currently classified. Yeasts are single-celled organisms, although some species with yeast forms may become mul-
ticellular through the formation of strings of connected budding
cells known as *pseudohyphae*, or *false hyphae*, as seen in most molds.

Zonulin: a protein that modulates the permeability of tight junctions
between cells of the wall of the digestive tract. Zonulin has been
implicated in the pathogenesis of Celiac disease and diabetes
mellitus type 1. It is being studied as a target for vaccine adjuvants.
Gliaden activates zonulin signaling irrespective of the genetic
expression of autoimmunity, leading to increased intestinal permeability to macromolecules.

NOTES

Welcome

1. I recently checked in with this friend, who contacted me for information on the autoimmune protocol. She is currently suffering from a couple different autoimmune conditions and has severe irritable bowel syndrome. She was diagnosed with a leaky gut and several food intolerances, including wheat and alcohol.

Chapter One: What the Frak Is HS?

1. "Supporting Hidradenitis Suppurativa Patients and Medical Research," *HS-USA*. http://HS-USA.org/

2. Ibid.

3. J. von der Werth, H.C. Williams. "The natural history of hidradenitis suppurativa." *Journal of European Academy and Dermatology and Venereology*. 2000 Sep;14(5):389-92.

4. Ibid.

5. Ibid.

6. Ibid.

7. M. Nazary, H. van der Zee, E.P. Prens, et al. "Pathogenesis and pharmacotherapy of Hidradenitis suppurativa." *European Journal of Pharmacology*. 2011 Dec;672(1-3):1-8.

8. Ibid.

9. H.H. van der Zee, C.J. van der Woude, et al. "Hidradenitis suppurativa and inflammatory bowel disease: are they associated? Results of a pilot study." *British Journal of Dermatology*. 2010 Jan;162(1):195-7.

10. A great example that correlation is not causation.

11. H. van der Zee, et al. "Hidradenitis suppurativa and inflammatory bowel disease: are they associated? Results of a pilot study."

12. "Supporting Hidradenitis Suppurativa Patients and Medical Research," *HS-USA*.

13. "Basic Statistics," *Center for Disease Control and Prevention*. 2011. http://www.cdc.gov/hiv/topics/surveillance/basic.htm

14. H. Hurley, Ed., R. Roenigk, H. Roenigk, "Axillary hyperhidrosis, apocrine bromhidrosis, hidradenitis suppurativa, and familial benign pemphigus: surgical approach." *Dermatologic Surgery* (Marcel Dekker:

New York, 1989), 729–739.

15. J. von der Werth, "Hidradenitis suppurativa." *Dermatology in Practice*. 2001;9(3):1-3.

16. Ibid. 2.

17. Mayo Clinic, "Hidradenitis Suppurativa Symptoms." http://www.mayoclinic.com/health/hidradenitis-suppurativa/DS00818/DSECTION=symptoms

Chapter Two: What the Doctors Will Tell You
1. "Supporting Hidradenitis Suppurativa Patients and Medical Research." *HS-USA*. http://HS-USA.org/

2. R. Drucker, *The Code of Life*. 2008. Accessed online at www.thecodeoflife.info. 76

3. *Dictionary.com*.

4. C. Kresser. "Naturally Get Rid of Acne by Fixing Your Gut." http://chriskresser.com/naturally-get-rid-of-acne-by-fixing-your-gut

5. J. von der Werth, "Hidradenitis suppurativa." *Dermatology in Practice*. 2001;9(3):2.

6. Ibid.

7. J. von der Werth, H.C. Williams, "The natural history of hidradenitis suppurativa." *Journal of European Academy and Dermatology and Venereology. JEADV.* 2000 Sep;14(5):389-92.

8. Y. Vandenplas, O. Brunser, H. Szajewska, "Saccharomyces boulardii in childhood." *Eurupean Journal of Pediatry.* 2009 March;168(3):253-65.

9. E. Dinleyici, M. Eren, N. Dogan, et al. "Clinical efficacy of Saccharomyces boulardii or metronidazole in symptomatic children with Blastocystis hominis infection." *Parasitology Research*. 2011 March;108(3):541-5.

10. T. Gerstmar, "Antibiotics and Leucopenia (low white blood cells)–Post 18; Day 18." October 11, 2011. http://www.aspirenaturalhealth.com/antibiotics-and-leukopenia-low-white-blood-cells-post-18-day-18-by-dr-tim-gerstmar-10112011/

11. J. von der Werth, "Hidradenitis suppurativa." 2001. p. 2.

12. *The Free Medical Dictionary*. http://medical-dictionary.thefreedictionary.com/Systemic+Corticosteroids

13. Ibid.

14. H. van der Zee, L. De Ruiter, D. van den Broecke, et al. "Elevated levels of tumour necrosis factor (TNF)-α, interleukin (IL)-1β and IL-10 in hidradenitis suppurativa skin: a rational for targeting TNF-α and IL-1β." *British Journal of Dermatology*. 2011 Jun;164(6):1292-8.

15. Ibid.

16. L. Walsh, G. Trinchieri, H. Waldorf, et al. "Human dermal mast cells contain and release tumor necrosis factor alpha, which induces endothelial leukocyte adhesion molecule 1." *Proceedings of the National Academy of Sciences of the United States of America*. 1991 May;88(10): 4220–4.

17. H. van der Zee, L. De Ruiter, D. van den Broecke, et al. "Elevated levels of tumour necrosis factor (TNF)-α, interleukin (IL)-1β and IL-10 in hidradenitis suppurativa skin: a rational for targeting TNF-α and IL-1β." *British Journal of Dermatology*. 2011 Jun;164(6):1292-8.

18. Ibid.

19. "Tumor Necrosis Factor-alpha (TNFα) Blockers: Label Change - Boxed Warning Updated for Risk of Infection from Legionella and Listeria," *FDA Official Website*. 2011 Sept. http://www.fda.gov

20. D. Adams, K. Gordon, A. Devenyi, M. Ioffreda, "Severe hidradenitis suppurativa treated with infliximab infusion." *JAMA Dermatology*. 2003 Dec;139(12):1540-2.

21. "How Pain Meds, Dysbiosis and Antibiotics Can Cause Leaky Gut." *Integrative Wellness*. 2011 Apr. http://integrativewellness.wordpress.com/2011/04/29/how-pain-meds-dysbiosis-and-antibiotics-can-cause-leaky-gut-syndrome/

22. M. Trescott, *AutoImmune Paleo*. http://www.autoimmunepaleo.wordpress.com

23. "What are Th1 Cytokines?" *Wise Geek*, http://www.wisegeek.com/what-are-th1-cytokines.htm

24. P. Goldsmith, P. Dowd, "Successful therapy of the follicular occlusion triad in a young woman with high dose oral antiandrogens and minocycline." *Journal of the Royal Society of Medicine*. 1993 Dec;(86):729-730.

25. Ibid.

26. R. Sitruk-Ware, A. Nath, "Metabolic effects of contraceptive steroids," *Review of Endocrine Metabolic Disorders*. 2011 Jun;12(2):63-75.

27. J. Brown, C. Farquar, O. Lee, et al. "Spironolactone versus placebo

or in combination with steroids for hirsutism and/or acne," *Cochrane database of systematic reviews*. 2009 Apr 15;(2):CD000194.

28. J. von der Werth "Hidradenitis suppurativa." *Dermatology in Practice*. 1-3.

29. Ibid.

30. Ibid.

31. Ibid.

Chapter Three: Autoimmunity 101

1. A. Fasano, "Surprises From Celiac Disease," *Scientific American*. 2009 August, 54.

2. L. Cordain, "Hidradenitis Suppurativa," *The Paleo Diet*. http://thepaleodiet.com/part-i-hidradenitis-suppurativa-and-the-paleo-diet/

3. H. H. van der Zee, et al. "Elevated levels of tumour necrosis factor (TNF)-α, interleukin (IL)-1β and IL-10 in hidradenitis suppurativa skin: a rational for targeting TNF-α and IL-1β." *British Journal of Dermatology*.

4. L. Cordain, "Hidradenitis Suppurativa," *The Paleo Diet*. http://thepaleodiet.com/part-i-hidradenitis-suppurativa-and-the-paleo-diet/

5. "Leaky Gut Syndrome," *Digestaqure*. http://www.digestaqure.com/Leaky-Gut-Syndrome.html

6. L. Cordain, *The Paleo Diet: Lose Weight and Get Healthy by Eating the Foods You Were Designed to Eat* (Hoboken, New Jersey: John Wiley & Sons, 2011), 94.

7. R. Drucker, "The Autoimmune Solution," 2011. http://www.thecodeoflife.info/dr.drucker/autoimmunity/my_direct_experience/the_solution/

8. L. Cordain, *The Paleo Diet: Lose Weight and Get Healthy by Eating the Foods You Were Designed to Eat*, 93.

9. "Skin," *National Geographic*. http://science.nationalgeographic.com/science/health-and-human-body/human-body/skin-article/

10. L. Cordain, *The Paleo Diet: Lose Weight and Get Healthy by Eating the Foods You Were Designed to Eat*, 93.

11. R. Drucker, "The Autoimmune Solution," *The Code of Life*. 2011, http://www.thecodeoflife.info/dr.drucker/autoimmunity/my_direct_experience/the_solution/

12. Better known autoimmune conditions include: diabetes, celiac

disease, rheumatoid arthritis, psoriasis, multiple sclerosis, endometriosis, Hashimoto's, lupus, narcolepsy, and restless leg syndrome, but that is just the tip of the iceberg. For a list with over two hundred autoimmune diseases, visit www.aarda.org.

13. R. Wolf, "Paleo Diet, Inflammation and Metformin," Mar., 2012, http://robbwolf.com/2012/03/09/paleo-diet-inflammation-metformin/

14. C. Kresser. "Pioneering Researcher Alessio Fasano MD on Gluten, Autoimmunity and Leaky Gut." Aug., 2012, http://chriskresser.com/pioneering-researcher-alessio-fasano-m-d-on-gluten-autoimmunity-leaky-gut

15. L. Cordain, *The Paleo Diet: Lose Weight and Get Healthy by Eating the Foods You Were Designed to Eat*, 93.

16. Ibid.

17. R. Wolf. *The Paleo Solution: The Original Human Diet.* (Victory Belt Publishing: Las Vegas, NV, 2010), 91.

18. Ibid.

19. L. Cordain, *The Paleo Diet: Lose Weight and Get Healthy by Eating the Foods You Were Designed to Eat.*

20. C.A. Wallace, "Arthritis Remission Criteria," *Childhood Arthritis and Rheumatology Research Alliance (CARRA)*, http://www.arthritistoday.org/conditions/juvenile-arthritis/all-about-ja/juvenile-arthritis-remission.php

21. "Autoimmune Disease and RA: Understanding the role played by the body's immune system in the progress of rheumatoid arthritis." *WedMD*. http://www.webmd.com/rheumatoid-arthritis/features/autoimmune-disease-and-ra

22. "Arthritis Remission Criteria." *Arthritis Today.* http://stage.arthritistoday.org/conditions/juvenile-arthritis/all-about-ja/arthritis-remission-criteria.php

23. Ibid.

24. R. Drucker. "The Autoimmune Solution." 2011. http://www.thecodeoflife.info/dr.drucker/autoimmunity/my_direct_experience/the_solution/

25. L. Cordain, *The Paleo Diet: Lose Weight and Get Healthy by Eating the Foods You Were Designed to Eat.*

Chapter Four: Follow Your Gut

1. C. Kresser, "Naturally Get Rid of Acne By Fixing Your Gut." http://chriskresser.com/naturally-get-rid-of-acne-by-fixing-your-gut

2. H. Van der Zee, L. de Ruiter, D. van den Broecke, et al. "Elevated levels of tumour necrosis factor (TNF)-α, interleukin (IL)-1β and IL-10 in hidradenitis suppurativa skin: a rational for targeting TNF-α and IL-1β." *British Journal of Dermatology.* 2011 Jun;164(6):1292-8.

3. M. Trescott, "Autoimmune Paleo." http://autoimmunepaleo.wordpress.com

4. C. Kresser, Feb 2011. "9 Steps to Perfect Health: #5 Heal Your Gut." http://chriskresser.com/9-steps-to-perfect-health-5-heal-your-gut

5. K. Brown, D. DeCoffe, E. Molcan, et al. "Diet-induced dysbiosis of the intestinal microbiota and the effects on immunity and disease." *Nutrients.* 2012 August; 4(8): 1095-1119.

6. L. Dethlefsen, D. Relman, "Incomplete recovery and individualized responses of the human distal gut microbiota to repeated antibiotic perturbation." 2010 Aug. Department of Microbiology and Immunology and Department of Medicine, Stanford University School of Medicine, Stanford CA and Veterans Affairs Palo Alto Health Care System, Palo Alto CA.

7. C. Kresser. "9 Steps to Perfect Health: #5 Heal Your Gut."

8. Get throat infections often? You may have mouth/throat flora dysbiosis. Gargle with probiotics before bed. Acid reflux? Drink yours mixed with water. Yeast infections? Dysbiosis of the vagina. Douche with a mixture of saline and water-soluble probiotics. Sinus infections or allergies? Add them to your neti pot. Lazy colon? I have two words for you: probiotic enema. Have fun!

9. S. Ballantyne, "What Is A Leaky Gut and How Can It Cause So Many Health Issues." March 2012. http://paleoparents.com/featured/guest-post-by-the-paleo-mom-what-is-a-leaky-gut

10. Ibid.

11. C. Kresser. "9 Steps to Perfect Health: #5 Heal Your Gut."

12. J. Visser, J. Rozing, A. Sapone, et al. "Tight Junctions, Intestinal Permeability, and Autoimmunity: Celiac Disease and Type 1 Diabetes Paradigms." *Annals of the New York Academy of Sciences.* 2009 May; 1165:195-205.

13. C. Kresser. Feb 2011.

14. S. Ballantyne. "How Do Grains, Legumes and Dairy Cause A Leaky Gut. Part 1: Lectins." March 2012. http://www.thepaleomom. com/2012/03/how-do-grains-legumes-and-dairy-cause.html

15. L. Cordain. "Loren Cordain – Autoimmune Disease and Food Triggers." *Me And My Diabetes.* Nov 2011. http://www.meandmydiabetes. com/2011/11/30/loren-cordain-autoimmune-disease-and-food-triggers/

16. J. O'Keefe Jr, L. Cordain, "Cardiovascular disease resulting from a diet and lifestyle at odds with our Paleolithic genome: how to become a 21st-century hunter-gatherer." *Mayo Clinic Proceedings.* 2004 Jan;79(1):101-8.

17. L. Kowalski, J. Bujko, "Evaluation of biological and clinical potential of Paleolithic diet." [Translated from Polish] *Rocz Panstw Zaki Hig.*2012; 63(1):9-15.

18. S. Ballantyne. "How Do Grains, Legumes and Dairy Cause A Leaky Gut. Part 1: Lectins." 2012. http://paleoparents.com/featured/ how-do-grains-legumes-and-dairy-cause-a-leaky-gut-part-1-lectins/

19. I.M. Vasconcelos, J.T. Oliveira, "Antinutritional properties of plant lectins." *Toxicon.* 2004 Sep 15;44(4):385-403.

20. L. Cordain, L. Toohey, M.J. Smith, et al. "Modulation of immune function by dietary lectins in rheumatoid arthritis." *British Journal of Nutrition.* 2000 Mar;83(3):207-17.

21. A. Pusztai, "Dietary lectins are metabolic signals for the gut and modulate immune and hormone functions." *European Journal of Clinical Nutrition.* 1993 Oct;47(10):691-9.

22. G. Sarwar Gilani, C. Wu Xiao, K.A. Cockell, "Impact of antinutritional factors in food proteins on the digestibility of protein and the bioavailability of amino acids and on protein quality." *British Journal of Nutrition.* 2012 Aug;108 Suppl 2:S315-32.

23. I.E. Liener, "Implications of antinutritional components in soybean foods." *Critical Review Food Science Nutrition.* 1994;34(1):31-67.

24. L. Cordain. Nov 2011.

25. S. Guyenet, "How To Eat Grains." Jan 2009. http://wholehealth-source.blogspot.com/2009/01/how-to-eat-grains.html

26. J.M. Gee, J.M. Wal, K. Miller, et al. "Effect of saponin on the transmucosal passage of beta-lactoglobulin across the proximal small intestine of normal and beta-lactoglobulin sensitized rats." *Toxicology.*

1997 Feb;117(2-3):219-28.

27. C. Kresser, http://chriskresser.com/naturally-get-rid-of-acne-by-fixing-your-gut.

28. A.C. Chao, J.V. Nguyen, M. Broughall, et al. Enhancement of intestinal model compound transport by DS-1, a modified Quillaja saponin. *Journal of Pharmacology Science*. 1998 Nov;87(11):1395-9.

29. Ibid.

30. Ibid.

31. K. Yu, F. Chen, C. Li, Absorption, disposition and pharmacokinetics of saponins from Chinese medicinal herbs. *Curr. Drug Metab*. 2012 Jun 1;13(5):577-98.

32. L. Cordain, blog.

33. N. Quinn, "Why No Grains & Legumes (and nuts?): Phytates." April 2011. http://www.paleoplan.com/2011/04-27/phytates/

34. W. Davis, *Wheat Belly* (New York: Rodale Inc., 2011), 39.

35. Ibid.

36. A. Brocard, A.C. Knol, A. Khammari, et al. "Hidradenitis suppurativa and zinc: a new therapeutic approach. A pilot study." *Dermatology*. 2007; 214(4):325-7.

37. N. Quinn, Apr 2011.

38. G. Famularo, "Probiotic lactobacilli: an innovative tool to correct the malabsorption syndrome of vegetarians?" *Medical Hypotheses*. 2005 65(6):1132-5.

39. L. Cordain, "Hidradenitis Suppurativa." http://thepaleodiet.com/part-i-hidradenitis-suppurativa-and-the-paleo-diet/

40. S. Ballantyne, "The Why's Behind the Autoimmune Protocol: Nightshades." Aug 2012. http://www.thepaleomom.com/2012/08/the-whys-behind-autoimmune-protocol.html

41. S. Ballantyne, "How Do Grains, Legumes and Dairy Cause A Leaky Gut – Part 2: Saponins and Protease Inhibitors." March 2012. http://paleoparents.com/featured/how-do-grains-legumes-and-dairy-cause-a-leaky-gut-part-2-saponins-and-protease-inhibitors/

42. E.A. Maga, B.C. Weimer, J.D. Murray, "Dissecting the role of milk components on gut microbiota composition." *Gut Microbes*. 2012 Dec 12;4(2).

43. L. Cordain, "Loren Cordain – Autoimmune Disease and Food Triggers." Nov 2011. http://www.meandmydiabetes.com/2011/11/30/

loren-cordain-autoimmune-disease-and-food-triggers/

44. M. Sisson, *The Primal Blueprint 21-Day Total Body Transformation*. (Malibu, CA: Primal Nutrition Inc., 2011), 118.

45. B.C. Melnik, S.M. John, P. Carrera-Bastos, et al. "The impact of cow's milk-mediated mTORC1-signaling in the initiation and progression of prostate cancer." *Nutr Metab* (London). 2012 Aug 14;9(1): 74.

46. T.F. Ramezani, N. Moslehi, G. Asghari, et al. "Intake of dairy products, calcium, magnesium and phosphorus in childhood and age at menarche in the Tehran lipid and glucose study." *PLoS One*. 2013 Feb;8(2):e57696.

47. Ibid., 117.

48. S. Ballantyne, "The Whys Behind The Autoimmune Protocol – Eggs." 2012 Jun. http://www.thepaleomom.com/2012/06/whys-behind-autoimmune-protocol-eggs.html

49. L. Tomljenovic, C.A. Shaw, "Mechanisms of aluminum adjuvant toxicity and autoimmunity in pediatric populations." *Lupus*. 2012 Feb;21(2):223-30.

50. C. Kresser, "Answers to Your Burning Questions About Digestion." 2011 Nov. *The Healthy Skeptic Podcast*. http://chriskresser.com/answers-to-your-burning-questions-about-digestion.

51. The National Candida Center. "Candida Yeast Infection, Leaky Gut, Irritable Bowel and Food Allergies." 2007. http://www.nationalcandidacenter.com/leaky-gut/

52. H.S. Hussein, J.M. Brasel, "Toxicity, metabolism and impact of mycotoxins on humans and animals." *Toxicology*. 2001 Oct;167(2):101-134.

53. M.E. Zain, "Impact of mycotoxins on humans and animals." *Journal of Saudi Chemical Society*. 2011 Apr;15(2):129-144.

54. V.E. Garcia, F.M. De Loudres, T.H. Oswaldo, et al. "Influence of Saccharomyces boulardii on the intestinal permeability of patients with Crohn's disease in remission." *Scand J Gastroenterol*. 2008;43(7):842-8.

55. Y. Vandenplas, O. Brunser, H. Szajewska. "Saccharomyces boulardii in childhood." *Eur J Pediatr*. 2009 Mar;168(3):253-65.

56. B. Clement, *The Vitamin Myth Exposed* (Juno Beach, FL: Healthful Communications, Inc., 2007), Part 1, Chapter 1. http://www.organicconsumers.org/articles/article_3697.cfm

57. A.J. Batchelor, J.E. Compston JE, "Reduced plasma half-life of

radio-labelled 25-hydroxyvitamin D3 in subjects receiving a high-fibre diet." *Br J Nutr*. 1983 Mar;49(2):213-6

58. S. Guyenet, "Gluten Sensitivity: Celiac Disease is the Tip of the Iceberg." 2008 Dec. http://wholehealthsource.blogspot.com/2008/12/gluten-sensitivity-celiac-disease-is.html

59. R. Wolf, 2010, 272.

60. L. Cordain, Nov 2011. Autoimmune Disease and Food Triggers.

61. L. Cordain, 2011, 52.

62 Ibid.

63. L. Cordain, "Hidradenitis Suppurativa." http://thepaleodiet.com/part-i-hidradenitis-suppurativa-and-the-paleo-diet/

64. A. Brocard, A.C. Knol, A. Khammari, et al. "Hidradenitis suppurativa and zinc: a new therapeutic approach. A pilot study." *Dermatology*. 2007;214(4):325-7.

65. B. Dréno, A. Khammari, A. Brocard, et al. "Hidradenitis Suppurativa: The Role of Deficient Cutaneous Innate Immunity." *Arch Dermatol*. 2012;148(2):182-186.

66. D. Holmannova, M. Kolackova, J. Krejsek, "Vitamin C and its physiological role with respect to the components of the immune system." [Article in Czech] *Vnitr Lek*. 2012 Oct;58(10):743-9.

67. Ibid.

68. Ibid.

69. Ballantyne. March 2012.

70. L. Cordain, *The Paleo Diet: Lose Weight and Get Healthy by Eating the Foods You Were Designed to Eat* (Hoboken, New Jersey: John Wiley & Sons, 2011), 55.

71. Ibid.

Chapter Five: The Hormone Connection

1. R. Kelly, "Crohn's Disease and Your Period." June 2009. http://www.everydayhealth.com/blog/kelly-building-a-crohns-disease-community/crohns-disease-and-your-period/

2. E. Makrantonaki, C.C. Zouboulis, "Androgens and ageing of the skin." *Curr Opin Endocrinol Diabetes Obes.* 2009 Jun;16(3):240-5.

3. M. Cappel, D. Mauger, D, Thiboutot, "Correlation between serum levels of insulin-like growth factor 1, dehydroepiandrosterone sulfate and dihydrotestosterone and acne lesion counts in adult women." *Arch*

Dermatol. 2005 Mar;141(3):333-8.

4. P.S. Mortimer, R.P. Dawber, M.A. Gales, et al. "Mediation of hidradenitis suppurativa by androgens." *Br Med J* (Clin Red Ed). 1986 Jan 25;292(6515):245-8.

5. B.J. Harrison, G.F. Read, L.E. Hughes, "Endocrine basis for the clinical presentation of hidradenitis suppurativa." *Br J Surg.* 1988 Oct;75(10):972-5.

6. C.S. Negi, *Intro to Endocrinology* (New Delhi: PHI Learning Private Limited, 2009), 268.

7. T. Oosthuyse, A.N. Bosch, "The effect of the menstrual cycle on exercise metabolism." *Sports Med.* 2010 Mar 1;40(3):207-27.

8. Negi, 2009, 268.

9. Ibid.

10. T. Oosthuyse, 2010, 207-27.

11. D.M. Selva, G.L. Hammond, "Thyroid hormones act indirectly to increase sex hormone binding globulin production by liver via hepatocyte nuclear factor-4alpha." *J Mol Endocrinol.* 2009 Jul;43(1):19-27.

12. X. Wang, D.M. Keenan, S.M. Pincus, et al. "Oscillations in joint synchrony of reproductive hormones in healthy men." *Am J Physiol Endocrinol Metab.* 2011 Dec;301(6):E1163-73.

13. D.J. Moskovic, M.L. Eisenberg, L. I. Lipshultz. "Seasonal fluctuations in testosterone-estrogen ratio in men from the Southwest United States." *J Androl.* 2012 Nov-Dec;33(6):1298-304.

14. S. Kenouch, M. Lombes, F. Delahaye, et al. "Human skin as target for aldosterone: coexpression of mineralocorticoid receptors and 11 beta-hydroxysteroid dehydrogenase." *J Clin Endocrinol Metab.* 1994 Nov;79(5):1334-41.

15. M. Volpe, S. Rubattu, D. Ganten, et al. "Dietary salt excess unmasks blunted aldosterone suppression and sodium retention in the stroke-prone phenotype of the spontaneously hypertensive rat." *J Hypertens.* 1993 Aug;11(8):793-8.

16. F. Akin, M. Bastemir, E. Alkis, "Effect of insulin sensitivity on SHBG levels in premenopausal versus postmenopausal obese women." *Adv Ther.* 2007 Nov-Dec;24(6):1210-20.

17. R. Simo, A. Barbosa-Desongles, C. Saez-Lopez, et al. "Molecular Mechanism of TNFα–Induced Down-Regulation of SHBG Expression." *Mol Endocrinol.* 2012 Mar;26(3):438-46.

18. R. Simo, A. Barbosa-Desongles, C. Hernandez, et al. "IL1β down-regulation of sex hormone binding globulin production by decreasing HNF-4α via MEK-1/2 and JNK MAPK pathways." *Mol Endocrinol.* 2012 Nov;26(11):1917-27.

19. D.M. Selva, G.L. Hammond, "Thyroid hormones act indirectly to increase sex hormone binding globulin production by liver via hepatocyte nuclear factor-4alpha."*J Mol Endocrinol.* 2009 Jul;43(1):19-27.

20. R. Rosedale. "Insulin and it's Metabolic Effects" (lecture presented at Designs for Health Institutes Boulderfest, August,1999).

21. Ibid.

22. V. Douard, R.P. Ferraris. "The Role of Fructose Transporters in Diseases Linked to Excessive Fructose Intake." *J Physio.* 2013 Jan 15;591(Pt 2):401-14.

23. Y. Rayssiguier, E. Gueux, W. Nowacki, et al. "High fructose consumption combined with low dietary magnesium intake may increase the incidence of the metabolic syndrome by inducing inflammation." *Magnes Res.* 2006 Dec;19(4):237-43.

24. N. Velickovic, A. Djordjevic, A. Vasiljevic, et al. "Tissue-specific regulation of inflammation by macrophage migration inhibitory factor and glucocorticoids in fructose-fed Wistar rats." *Br J Nutr.* 2013 Jan;3:1-10.

25. Ibid.

26. M. Soleimani, "Dietary fructose, salt absorption and hypertension in metabolic syndrome: towards a new paradigm." *Acta Physiol* (Oxf). 2011 Jan;201(1):55-62.

27. S. Ballantyne, *The Paleo Approach: Reverse Autoimmune Disease and Heal Your Body* (Victory Belt Publishing, 2013). Advanced copy, page number not confirmed at time of publishing. Chapter: The Link Between High Carbohydrate Diets and Inflammation.)

28. Ibid.

29. Ibid.

30. L. Cordain, 2011, 77.

31. S. Ballantyne, 2013.

32. L. Cordain, 2011, 84.

33. R. Rosedale, Lecture, August 1999.

34. I don't actually know if every single hormone in the human body can be traced back to insulin <u>within six</u> steps. If you would like to spend

several decades mapping out the human endocrine system and get back to me, I'd appreciate it.

35. L. Cordain, 2011, 84.

Chapter Six: Wound Care

1. J.M. Von der Werth, H.C. Williams , "The Natural History of Hidradenitis Suppurativa." *J Eur Acad Dermatol Venereol.* 2001;14(5): 389-392.

2. "Skin Problems and Treatments Health Center. Boils Topic Overview." *WebMD* 2008 Oct. http://www.webmd.com/skin-problems-and-treatments/tc/boils-topic-overview

3. Ibid.

4. J.M. von der Werth, H.C. Williams, "The Natural History of Hidradenitis Suppurativa." *J Eur Acad Dermatol Venereol.* 2001;14(5): 389-392.

5. Ibid.

6. L. Cordain, "Hidradenitis Suppurativa." http://thepaleodiet.com/part-i-hidradenitis-suppurativa-and-the-paleo-diet/

7. P. Grant, "Spearmint herbal tea has significant anti-androgen effects in polycystic ovarian syndrome. A randomized controlled trial." *Phytotherapy Research.* 2010 Feb;24(2):186–188.

8. Ibid.

9. M. Akdogan, M.N. Tamer, E. Cure, et al. "Effect of spearmint (*Mentha spicata Labiatae*) teas on androgen levels in women with hirsutism." *Phytother Res.* 2007 May;21(5):444-7.

10. L. Cordain, "Hidradenitis Suppurativa." http://thepaleodiet.com/part-i-hidradenitis-suppurativa-and-the-paleo-diet/

11. A. Brocard, A.C. Knol, A. Khammari, et al. "Hidradenitis suppurativa and zinc: a new therapeutic approach. A pilot study." *Dermatology.* 2007; 214(4):325-7

12. Ibid.

13. L. Cordain, "Hidradenitis Suppurativa." http://thepaleodiet.com/part-i-hidradenitis-suppurativa-and-the-paleo-diet/

14. B.T. Kurien, A. D'Souza, R.H. Scofield, "Heat-solubilized curry spice curcumin inhibits antibody-antigen interaction in in vitro studies: A possible therapy to alleviate autoimmune disorders." *Mol Nutr Food Res.* 2010 August 54(8);1202-1209.

15. J. Mercola, "The Sweet Golden Treat That Can Help Wipe Out Deadly MRSA." 2012 February. http://articles.mercola.com/sites/articles/archive/2012/02/20/the-natural-way-to-speed-wound-healing.aspx

16. J. Majtan, J. Bohova, M. Horniackova, et al. "Anti-biofilm effects of honey against wound pathogens proteus mirabilis and enterobacter cloacae." *Phytother Res*. 2013 Mar 11. Doi: 10.1002/ptr.4957

17. Ibid.

18. A.S. Boyd, "Ichthammol revisited." *Int J Dermatol*. 2010 Jul;49(7):757-60.

19. Y.S. Chan, L.N. Cheng, J.H. Wu, et al. "A review of the pharmacological effects of Arctium lappa (burdock)." *Inflammopharmacology*. 2011 Oct;19(5):245-54.

20. Ibid.

21. D. Li, J.M. Kim, Z. Jin, et al. "Prebiotic effectiveness of inulin extracted from edible burdock." *Anaerobe*. 2008 Feb;14(1):29-34.

22. A.V. Arjoon, C.V. Saylor, M. May, "In vitro efficacy of antimicrobial extracts against the atypical ruminant pathogen *Mycoplasma mycoides* subsp. *capri*." *BMC Complement Altern Med*. 2012 Oct 2;12:169.

23. L. Cordain, "Hidradenitis Suppurativa." http://thepaleodiet.com/part-i-hidradenitis-suppurativa-and-the-paleo-diet/

24. T. von Woedtke, B. Schlüter, P. Pflegel, et al. "Aspects of the antimicrobial efficacy of grapefruit seed extract and its relation to preservative substances contained." *Pharmazie* 1999;54 (6): 452–6. PMID 10399191.

25. H. Vermeulen, Ed., J.M. van Hattem, M.N. Storm-Versloot, et al. "Topical silver for treating infected wounds," Cochrane Database of Systematic Reviews 2007(1): CD005486. PMID 17253557

26. Department of Health and Human Services (HHS), Public Health Service (PHS), Food and Drug Administration (FDA). August, 1999. "Over-the-counter drug products containing colloidal silver ingredients or silver salts." *Federal Register* 64 (158): 44653–8. PMID 10558603

27. R. Nicolo, Speer Laboratories. Personal Correspondence to Kiley MacLeod. http://www.notdying.wordpress.com

28. Emuaid Official Website: http://emuaid.com/Ingredient-Glossary.html

29. S. Buyukozturk, A. Gelincik, F. Ozseker, et al. "Nigella sativa (black seed) oil does not affect the T-helper 1 and T-helper 2 type cytokine

production from splenic mononuclear cells in allergen sensitized mice."
J Ethnopharmacol. 2005 Sep 14;100(3):295-8.

Chapter Seven: Dealing With Stress

1. E. Simone, "Common Factors of Autoimmune Disease." 2013 March. http://drellensimonend.wordpress.com/2012/03/13/3-common-factors-of-autoimmune-disease/

2. Ibid.

3. S. Ballantyne, "How mood and gut health are linked." 2012 Feb. http://www.thepaleomom.com/2012/02/how-mood-and-gut-health-are-linked.html

4. C. Kresser, "Naturally Get Rid Of Acne." 2011 Dec.

5. J. Mercola, "Are Probiotics the New Prozac?" Mercola.com 2013 Jul 25.

6. J.A. Bravo, P. Forsythe, M.V. Chew, et al. "Ingestion of the Lactobacillus strain regulates emotional behavior and central GABA receptor expression in a mouse via the vagus nerve." *Proc Natl Acad Sci USA.* 2011 Sep 20;108)38):16050-5.

7. J. Mercola, "Are Probiotics the New Prozac?" Mercola.com 2013 Jul 25.

8. K. Tillisch, J. Labus, L. Kilpatrick, et al. "Consumption of fermented milk product with probiotic modulates brain activity." *Gastroenterology.* 2013 Jun;144(7):1394-401.

9. K. Brown, D. DeCoffe, E. Molcan, et al. "Diet-induced dysbiosis of the intestinal microbiota and the effects on immunity and disease." *Nutrients.* 2012 August;4(8):1095-1119.

10. N.A. Abreu, N.A. Nagalingam, Y. Song, et al. "Sinus Microbiome Diversity Depletion and Corynebacterium tuberculostearicum Enrichment Mediates Rhinosinusitis." *Sci Transl Med* 2012 Sep;4(151), p. 151.

11. I am not saying that proper hygiene doesn't have its place. After all, I certainly wouldn't want a doctor to operate on me without first scrubbing the everloving crap out of his hands. However, the use of antibacterial and antibiotic products is out of control in our society. It is weakening our immune systems and actually making us sicker. We evolved along with the bacteria on our skin, and in our eyes and nose—constantly killing them off does not seem to be doing us any favors.

12. M. Lamprecht, A. Frauwallner, "Exercise, intestinal barri-

er dysfunction and probiotic supplementation." *Med Sport Sci.* 2012 Oct;59:47-56

13. A. Paturel, "The 5 Health Benefits of Having An Orgasm." *Self Magazine Online*, September 2011. http://www.self.com/health/blogs/healthyself/2011/09/the-5-health-benefits-of-havin.html

Chapter Eight: Phase I: The Elimination Diet

1. V. Fassnacht, E. Reymond, "The Evolution of Allergies." *Cern Medical Service* PDF, 1.

2. Ibid.

3. L. Cordain, 2011, 82-3.

4. J. Reasoner, "Can Coconut Oil Really Help Me Heal My Gut?" *SCD Lifestyle.* 2010. http://scdlifestyle.com/2010/06/jordan's-scd-thoughts-from-the-kitchen-edition-2...-can-coconut-oil-really-help-me-heal-my-gut/

5. S. Guyenet, "Gluten Sensitivity: Celiac Disease is the Tip of the Iceberg." 2008 Dec. http://wholehealthsource.blogspot.com/2008/12/gluten-sensitivity-celiac-disease-is.html

6. C. Cannistra, V. Finocchi, A. Trivisonno, et al. "New perspectives in the treatment of Hidradenitis suppurativa: Surgery and brewer's yeast-exclusion diet." *Surgery.* 2013 Jul 25.

7. K. Monastyrsky, "Fiber Menace." 2008. Chapter 1, available online at http://www.fibermenace.com.

8. Ibid.

9. Ibid.

10. B. Patel, R. Schutte, P. Sporns, et al. "Potato glycoalkaloids adversely affect intestinal permeability and aggravate inflammatory bowel disease." *Inflammatory Bowel Disease.* 2002 Sep;8(5):340-6.

11. V. Iablokov, B.C. Sydora, R. Foshaug, et al. "Naturally occurring glycoalkaloids in potatoes aggravate intestinal inflammation in two mouse models of inflammatory bowel disease." *Dig Dis Sci.* 2010 Nov;55(11):3078-85

12. Wikipedia – Potato. http://en.wikipedia.org/wiki/Potato

13. J. Lachman, K. Hamouz, J. Musilova, et al. "Effect of peeling and three cooking methods on the content of selected phytochemicals in potato tubers with various colour of flesh." *Food Chemistry.* 2013 Jun. 138(2-3):1189-1197

14. I. Shaw, *Is it Safe to Eat? Enjoy Eating and Minimize Food Risks* (Berlin: Springer, 2005), 129.

15. V. Iablokov, et al. 2010 Nov.

16. H.H. Van der Zee, et al., 2011 Jun.

17. H.H. Van der Zee, J.D. Laman, L. de Ruiter, et al. "Adalimumab (antitumour necrosis factor-α) treatment of hidradenitis suppurativa ameliorates skin inflammation: an in situ and ex vivo study." *British Journal of Dermatology*. 2012 Feb;166(2):298-305.

18. S. Ballantyne, 2012 Aug.

19. L. Cordain, "Loren Cordain – Autoimmune Disease and Food Triggers." Nov 2011.

20. E. Koh, S. Kaffka, A.E. Mitchell. "A long-term comparison of the influence of organic and conventional crop management practices on the content of the glycoalkaloid α-tomatine in tomatoes." *Journal of Science, Food and Agriculture*. 2012 Oct 15;9999(9999).

21. A. Schwarz, E.C. Felippe, M.M. Bernardi, et al. "Impaired female sexual behavior of rat offspring exposed to Solanum lycocarpum unripe fruits during gestation and lactation: lack of hormonal and fertility alterations." *Pharmacol Biochem Behav*. 2005 Aug;81(4):928-34.

22. E. Jensen-Jarolim, L. Gajdzik, I. Haberl, et al. "Hot spices influence permeability of human intestinal epithelial monolayers." *Journal of Nutrition*. 1998 Mar;128(3):577-81.

23. M. Trescott, *The Autoimmune Paleo Cookbook*. 2013, p. 15

24. M.B. Abou-Donia, E.M. El-Masry, et al. "Splenda Alters Gut Microflora and Increases Intestinal P-Glycoprotein and Cytochrome P-450 in Male Rats." *Journal of Toxicology and Environmental Health* 2008, 71: 1415-1429

25. Ibid.

26. J. Mercola, K. Degen-Pearsall, *Sweet Deceptions: Why Splenda, NutraSweet and the FDA May Be Hazardous To Your Health* (Nashville, TN: Thomas Nelson, 2006), Chapter Four.

27. D.B. Mawhinney, R.B. Young, B.J. Vanderford, et al. "Artificial sweetener sucralose in U.S. drinking water systems." *Environ Sci Technol*. 2011 Oct 15;45(20):8716-22.

28. C. Cannistra, V. Finocchi, A. Trivisonno, et al. "New perspectives in the treatment of Hidradenitis suppurativa: Surgery and brewer's yeast-exclusion diet." *Surgery*. 2013 Jul 25

29. S. Wood, R. Pithadia, T. Rehman, et al. "Chronic alcohol exposure renders epithelial cells vulnerable to bacterial infection." *PLoS One.* 2013;8(1):e54646

30. S.H. Kim, F. Abbasi, C. Lamendola, et al. "Effect of moderate alcoholic beverage consumption on insulin sensitivity in insulin-resistant, nondiabetic individuals." *Metabolism.* 2009 Mar;58(3):387-92.

31. P. Chek, *How to Eat, Move and Be Healthy!* (San Diego, CA: CHEK Institute, 2004), 79.

32. J.A. Saunders, D.E. Blume, "Quantification of major tobacco alkaloids by high-performance liquid chromatography." *Journal of Chromatography.* 1981(205)147-154.

33. K.J. Clemens, S. Caille, L. Stinus, et al.. "The addition of five minor tobacco alkaloids increases nicotine-induced hyperactivity, sensitization and intravenous self-administration in rats." *The International Journal of Neuropyschopharmacology.* 2009 Nov;12(10):1355-66

34. National Digestive Diseases Information Clearinghouse. "Smoking and Your Digestive System." http://digestive.niddk.nih.gov/ddiseases/pubs/smoking/

35. G. Debry, *Coffee and Health.* (Paris: John Libbey Eurotext, 1994), 106.

36. R. Nagel, "Living With Phytic Acid." The Weston A. Price Foundation. 2010 March. http://www.westonaprice.org/food-features/living-with-phytic-acid

37. G. Debry, *Coffee and Health.* (Paris: John Libbey Eurotext, 1994), 106.

38. L. Cordain, "Hidradenitis Suppurativa." http://thepaleodiet.com/part-i-hidradenitis-suppurativa-and-the-paleo-diet/

39. M. Kleinewietfeld, A. Manzel, J. Titze, et al. "Sodium chloride drives autoimmune disease by the induction of pathogenic TH17 cells." *Nature.* 2013 Mar 6. doi: 10.1038/nature11868

40. S. Ballantyne, "Gluten Cross Reactivity: How Your Body Can Still Think You're Eating Gluten Even After Giving It Up." 2012 Oct. http://www.thepaleomom.com/2012/10/gluten-cross-reactivity-how-your-body-can-still-think-youre-eating-gluten-even-after-giving-it-up.html

41. hCG stands for Human Chorionic Gonadotropin, a hormone naturally produced by the placenta in pregnant women that controls

metabolism throughout the pregnancy. Followers of the hCG diet are injected with this hormone and are subjected to a very low calorie diet. Although the safety of this diet is controversial, proponents claim they are able to effectively lose weight on it.

42. S. Guyenet, "Celiac Disease is the Tip of the Iceberg." 2008 Dec. http://wholehealthsource.blogspot.com/2008/12/gluten-sensitivity-celiac-disease-is.html

Chapter Nine: Phase II: Reintroduction and Designing Your Personal Ancestral Diet

1. *23andMe.* Genetic Testing for Carrier Status, Disease Risk and Drug Response. https://www.23andme.com/health/drugs/

2. S. Roberts, "The Rise of Personal Science: Implications for Statistics," 2012 Tsinghua University and the University of California, Berkeley.

3. M. Sisson, *The Primal Blueprint* (Malibu CA: Primal Nutrition, Inc., 2009)14-15.

4. Western doctors tend to treat each symptom and/or body part individually, instead of the more holistic approach of looking at the whole body as a complete system. This type of "doctoring" resulted in **over 10 years** of doctor's appointments for me just to get a diagnosis of PCOS. I was prescribed dozens of drugs for the different **symptoms** of PCOS, but not a single doctor looked for the root cause. I ended up diagnosing myself.

5. L. Cordain, "Autoimmune Disease and Food Triggers," Nov 2011. http://www.meandmydiabetes.com/2011/11/30/loren-cordain-autoimmune-disease-and-food-triggers/

6. S. Ballantyne, "Reintroducing Foods After Following The Autoimmune Protocol," 2009 Sep. http://www.thepaleomom.com/2012/09/reintroducing-foods-after-following-the-autoimmune-protocol.html

7. Ibid.

8. S. Ballantyne, "How Long Does It Take The Gut To Repair After Gluten Exposure?" 2012 Sept. http://www.thepaleomom.com/2012/09/how-long-does-it-take-the-gut-to-repair-after-gluten-exposure.html

9. Ibid.

RECIPE INDEX

SUBJECT INDEX

A

Abscess, 17, **23**, 38, 43, 111, 114, 116, 261, 267

Accidental dosing, 192-196

Acid reflux, 61, 72, 77, 184

Acne, 3
  adult, 5-7
  conglobata, 22, 261, 265
  cystic, 5, 19, 38, 116, 148
  inversa, 261

Acne medications, 38-9, 44

Adjuvant, 78-9, 85, 161, 276

Aldosterone, 32, 44, 97, 99, **101-2**, 261

Alkaloids, 43, 75, **80-81**, 85, 162-67, 169, 176, 261, 266

Allergy, 82, 132, 148, 184, 195, 244

Amino acids, 73, 105

Anabolic steroid, 97, 99

Androgen, 42, 44, 97-98, 103, 162

Anemia, 61, 79, 80, 273

Ancestral diet. *See also Primal and Paleo.* 2, 102-110, 117, 146, 149, 161, 178, **180-202**

Antacids, 85

Antiandrogens. *See also Birth Control Pills.* 42

Antibacterial, 7, 30, 91, 112, 114, 117-19, 121, 123, 125-26, 158, 261, 262

Antibiotics,
  and gut flora, 85, 89
  and yeast overgrowth, 86-87

as treatment, 3, 5-8, 11, 18, 28, 30, **33-38**, 45, 72, 79, 235, 237-38, 240-41, 244
  in food, 151, 193

Antibodies, 42, 59, 67-8, 78, 82, 262

Antidepressant, 8, 132

Antifungal, 121, 126, 262

Antimicrobial, 82, 114, 116, 121-23, 126, 153, 262

Antinutrients. *See also specific types.* 75-76, 83, 88, 93, 149, 175-77, 229, 262, 265, 271

Anus, 68, 72, 269, 271

Apocrine glands, 19, 31, 57, 58, 263, 267

Armpits, 17, 19, 22-24, 56-57, 74, 122, 243, 263

Arthritis, 20, 40, 55, 60-63, 66, 81-2, 96, 234

Aspirin. *See also NSAIDs.* 39, 271

Asthma, 40, 59, 70, 96, 264

Auto-antibodies, 84

Autoimmune/autoimmunity, 2, 6, 10-11, 30, 33-37, 40, **55-67**, 70, 75, 77, 81, 82, 84, 88, 91, 102, 110, 120, 129-31
  cycles, 65
  diet/protocol, 2, 3, 11, 94, 141, **142-196**, 231-34, 239-43, 245
  leaky gut, 69-87
  Neolithic foods, 74-79
  response, 11, 34, 45, 72, 76, 85, 92, 93, 132, 234,

Axillae, 17

immune, 35, 57, 73-74, 76, 91, 130, 267, 275
macrophage 57, 270
memory, 67
skin, 90, 99, 102, 135,
T (TH17), 177, 270
Cigarettes. *See also Tobacco.* 167
Circulatory system, 68, 73-74, 76, 86, 264, 269
Childhood Arthritis and Rheumatology Research Alliance (CARRA), 66
Code of Life, The, 41, 60-62
Coffee, **175-76**, 178, 185-86, 191, 203, 215
Cold laser therapy, 46
Colloidal silver, **126-127**
Colon, 61-62, 265, 269
Constipation, 34, 69, 72, 86, 93, 184
Cordain, Loren, 57-58, 60-61, 63, 67, 75, 83, 93, 122, 176, 242, 247, 255, 257
Corn, 78, 88, 106-07, 119, 140, 151, 153, 155, 160, 167, 168-69, 173, 193-95, 220, 237-38
Cortisol, 97, 99, 101-102, 107, 109, 134-35, 139, 264, 273-74
Cortisone, 40, 87, 109
Corticosteroids, 39-40, 87, 261, 274
Corticotropin-Releasing Hormone (CRH), 40, 264
Cryotherapy. *See Cold Laser Therapy.*
Cramps, 26, 44, 72, 81
Crohn's disease, 20, 61, 91, 96, 167

Cures, 62, 117
Cyst, 3, 5, 9, 19, 38, 43, 116, 148, 265, 274
Cytokines, 35, 37, 40-42, 57, 71, 91, 103, 107-08, 130, 136, 163, 263-64, 275

D

DNA, 158, 165, 181, 273
Dairy, 9, 63, 75, 81-83, 87, 150, 155, 158, 162, 172, 176, 179, 183, 186-87, 189, 191-93, 195, 202, 228, 237-38, 242, 244, 274
Dandruff, 2, 58, 117, 184
Davis, William, 77, 256
Deep breathing and meditation, 138
Dendritic cells. *See cells.*
Deodorant, 7, 117
Depression, 5, 20, 26, 34, 38, 40, 70, 77, 101, 130-31, 184, 264
Dermal, 68, 99
Dermatitis herpetiformis, 60-61
Dermatologists, 6, 8, 17, 19, 38, 68
Diabetes, 2, 20, 59-61, 63, 70, 75, 88, 93, 99, 103, 108, 120, 234, 264, 266, 268, 270, 276
Diarrhea, 34-35, 69, 72, 81, 89, 157, 176, 184, 262
Diet,
American, 76, 104, 274
ancestral, 2
autoimmune, 3, 11, 231-32, 239
elimination. S*ee elimination diet.*